Comfort Soups and Stews

30 Indulgent Gluten-Free and Vegan Recipes

GRUBB
BLACKWOOD
PUBLISHING

DEDICATION

This book is written in loving memory of my dad who went to sleep
February 9, 2019
He was a firm believer in education as a vehicle to better oneself. He was also a hard worker and a giver. He would give the shirt off his back for his loved ones and strangers. These qualities have laid the foundation for me to always keep growing, learning and sharing my gifts to benefit others.

INTRODUCTION

Here's the perfect Cookbook for Gluten-Free Vegan Soup And Stews. Transition easily to eating healthier with these 30 flavorful and easy to prepare recipes, from French onion soup, Italian Tuscan Soup and Black Bean And Butternut Squash Stew.

The Gluten-Free Vegan Soup And Stews Cookbook filled with plenty of recipes for people who are transitioning from eating, animal meat, dairy, eggs, wheat, barley, and rye.
The cookbook has 30 colorful photos of each recipe with step by step instructions. A shopping list and helpful tips.

Whether you are just exploring a new way of eating, trying to increase your consumption of fruit and vegetables or just adding more recipes to your repertoire, this cookbook has a variety of tasty soups and stews just for you.
These tried and tested recipes will take your plant-based lifestyle to the next level!

CONTENT

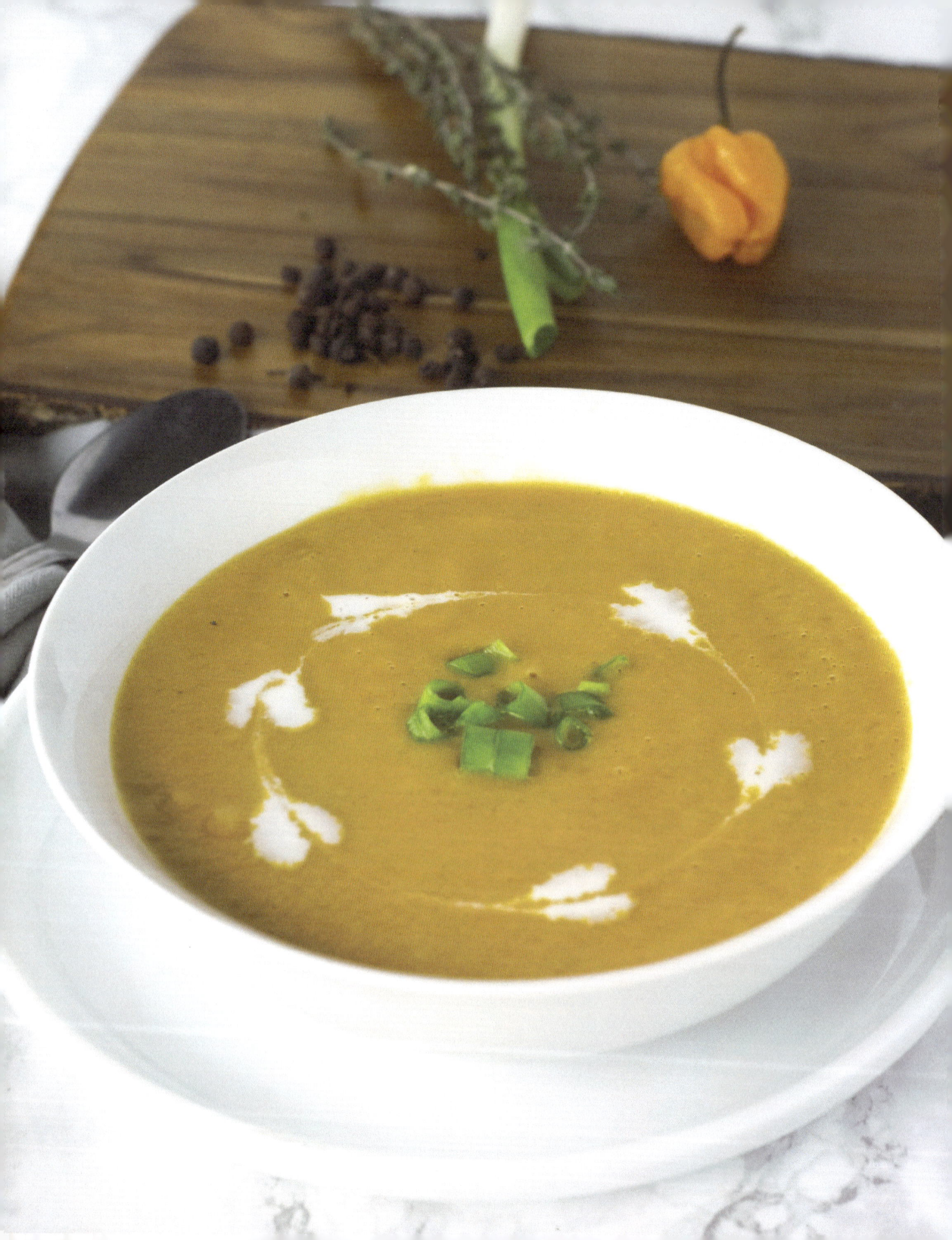

JAMAICAN PUMPKIN SOUP (PUREED)

This Jamaican Pumpkin Soup is an adapted version of the Jamaican-style pumpkin soup without any meat. Pumpkin soup was my family's favorite when growing up, which my mom made weekly. Enjoy the taste of the Tropics with this delicious and easy to prepare soup!

INGREDIENTS

- 2 tablespoons coconut oil, or water
- 1 cup onion, minced
- 3 cloves garlic, minced
- 1/4 cup celery, chopped
- 2 green onions, chopped, extra for garnish
- 1 tablespoon fresh parsley, finely chopped or 1 teaspoon dried
- 1 sprig fresh thyme, 1/4 teaspoon dried
- 4 cups Jamaican Pumpkin, peeled and cut into chunks
- 1 cup potato, peeled and chopped
- 1 cup carrot, diced
- 4 cups vegetable broth, (or 2 vegetable bouillon plus 4 cups water)
- 1/2 cup coconut milk, extra for garnish
- 1 whole Scotch Bonnet pepper, or 1/4 teaspoon cayenne pepper
- 1/4 teaspoon ground allspice, (optional)
- salt, to taste

INSTRUCTIONS

1. Heat the oil in a large pot, add onion and garlic and saute for 4 minutes until onion is soft. Add celery and carrot, and cook until celery is soft or for about 3 minutes.

2. Add green onion, parsley, thyme, pumpkin, potato, stock, coconut milk, pepper, and allspice.

3. Bring to boil, reduce heat to simmer and cook for 30 minutes. Remove the Scotch Bonnet pepper and thyme sprigs.

4. Cool slightly, puree the soup in batches using a blender or a stick blender. Season with salt to your taste.

5. Serve in bowls garnished with coconut milk and spring onions.

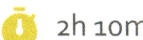 2h 10m   6

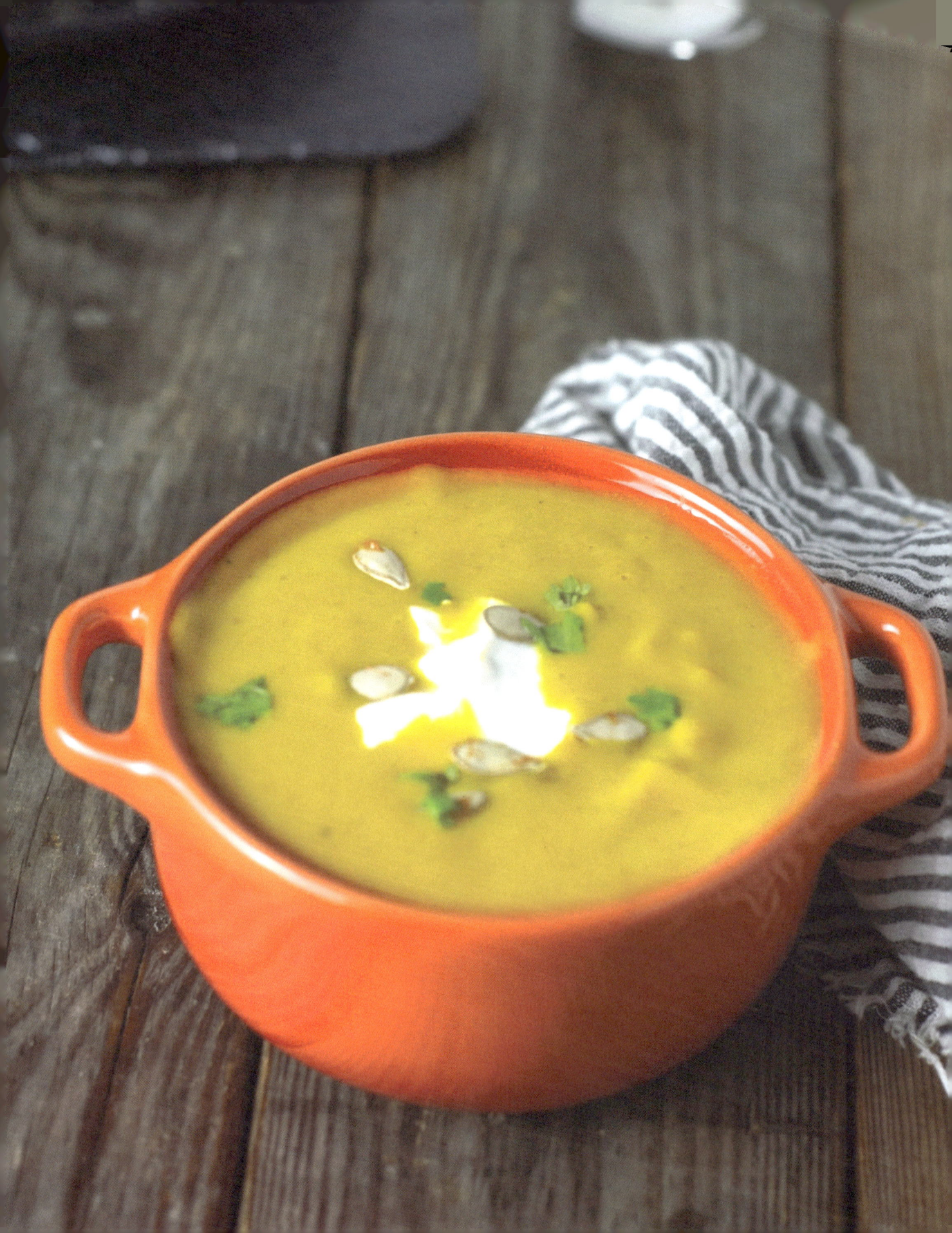

BUTTERNUT SQUASH SOUP

This is a creamy yet well-spiced butternut squash soup that just feels like comfort. This is a recreation of the Panera Bread autumn squash, but without any dairy ingredients.

INGREDIENTS

- 1 yellow onion, medium
- 2 lbs butternut squash, cubed
- 2 carrots, chopped
- ½ cup pumpkin puree
- 4 cups vegetable broth
- 2 cups apple juice
- 1 teaspoon curry powder
- ½ teaspoon ground cinnamon
- pinch of cardamom
- pinch of nutmeg
- 2 tablespoon coconut oil
- ¼ cup vegan cream cheese
- ¼ cup non-dairy milk
- 2 tablespoon organic cane sugar
- salt, to taste

INSTRUCTIONS

1. In a large pot over medium-low heat, add coconut oil and saute onions until soft.

2. Add squash, carrots, pumpkin, vegetable broth, apple juice, and spices to pot.

3. Bring to a boil, then reduce heat to low and simmer for 20 minutes.

4. Add coconut oil, cream cheese, milk, sugar, and salt to taste. Use an immersion blender, or blend in batches until creamy.

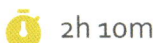 2h 10m   6

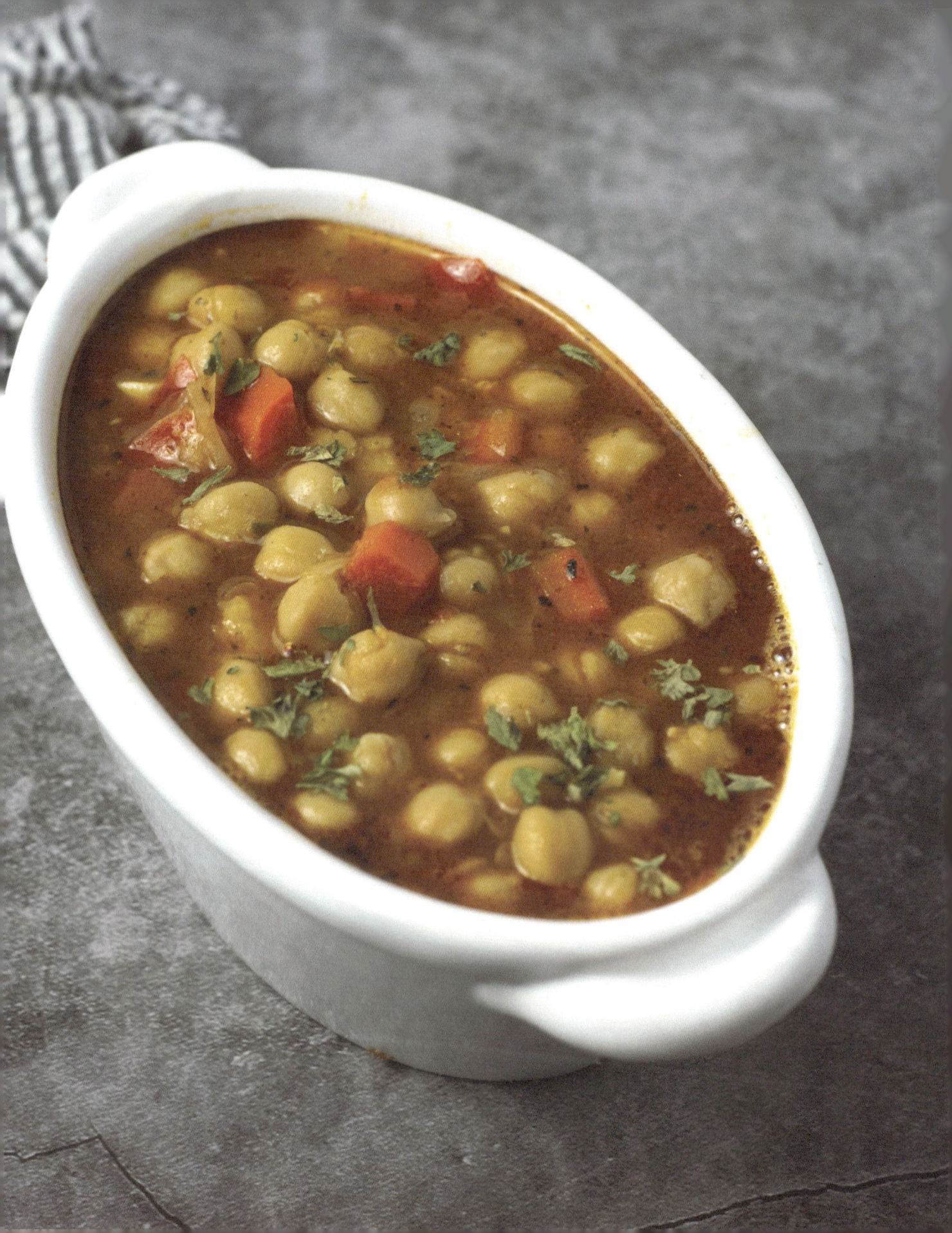

CHICKPEA STEW

Here is the best comforting and hearty chickpea stew ever! Made with simple ingredients from basic ingredients with an amazingly delicious taste that will keep you coming back for more!

INGREDIENTS

- 2 (15 ounce) cans chickpeas
- 1 tablespoon olive oil
- 1 medium onion, minced
- 2 cloves garlic, minced
- ¼ cup red bell pepper, chopped
- 1 medium tomato, chopped
- 1 carrot, diced
- 1 teaspoon dried parsley
- ½ teaspoon dried basil
- ½ tsp dried oregano
- 1 tablespoon tomato paste
- 2 cups vegetable broth
- ½ teaspoon salt
- ¼ teaspoon cayenne powder

INSTRUCTIONS

1. Drain chickpeas and reserve 2 cups of the broth and set aside.

2. Heat oil or water in a large saucepan on medium-high heat. Add onions and cook until soft, or for about 4 minutes.

3. Add garlic and cook for 30 seconds stirring. Add bell pepper, tomatoes, carrots, chickpeas, parsley, basil and oregano.

4. Add tomato paste and vegetable broth or reserved chickpeas broth, cover saucepan and bring to boil. Reduce to a simmer for 20-30 minutes or until thickened.

5. Mash some of the chickpeas, with the back of a fork to thicken stew.

6. Check seasoning, add cayenne pepper and extra salt and pepper as needed.

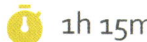 1h 15m 6

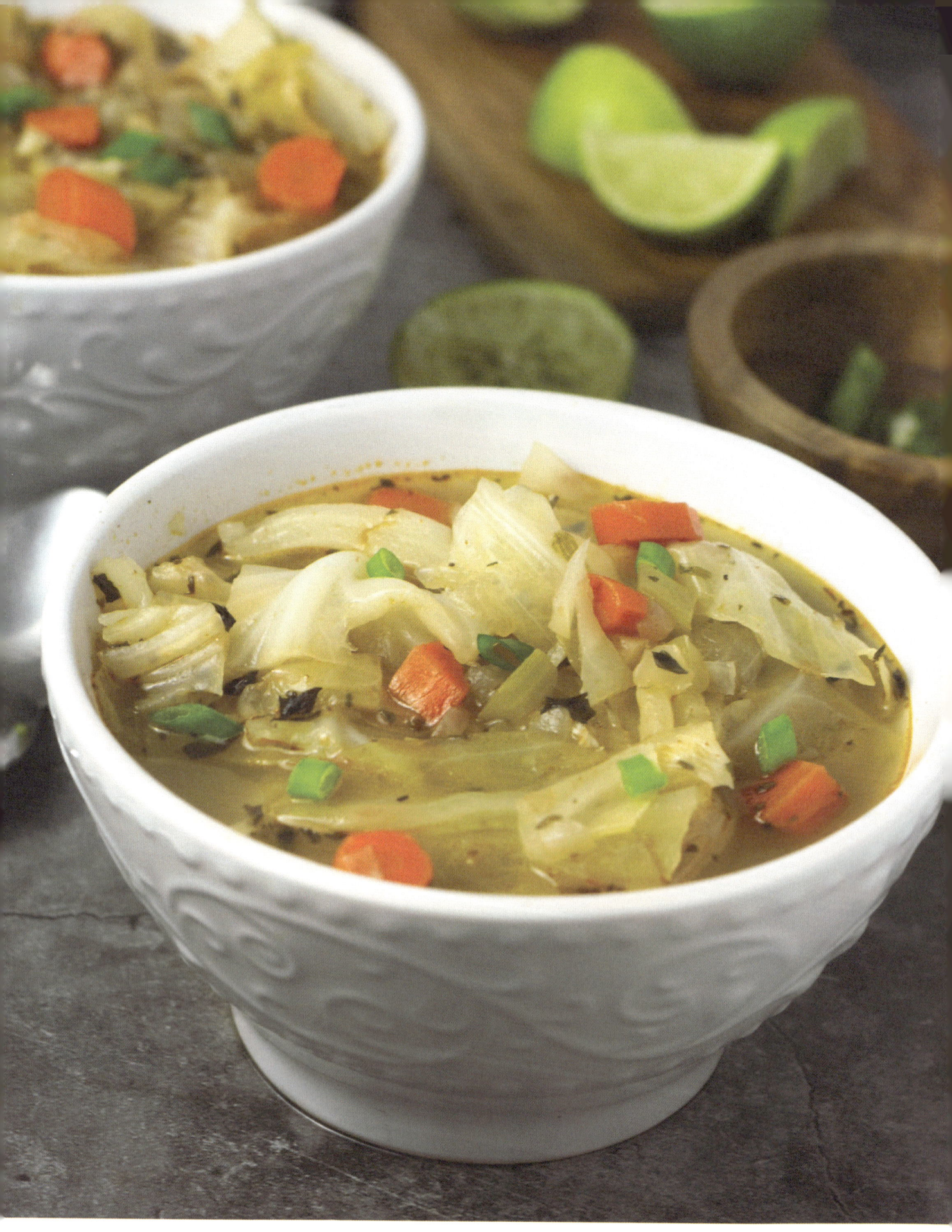

VEGAN CABBAGE SOUP

After the Thanksgiving and Christmas festivities are over and we have gained a few extra pounds. I have the perfect solution to help us shed those unwanted pounds! It is my very delicious vegan, vegetarian cabbage soup.

INGREDIENTS

- 1 tbsp olive oil, (or 1/4 cup water for sauteing)
- 1 medium onion, finely chopped
- 3 cloves garlic, minced
- 2 stalks celery, chopped
- 2 green onions, chopped (white & green parts)
- 2 carrots, cut in circles
- 2 sprigs fresh thyme, or 1 teaspoon dried
- 1 tsp parsley flakes
- 1 tsp dried basil
- 1 lb green cabbage, roughly chopped
- 2 quarts vegetable broth1/2 tsp paprika
- 1/4 tsp Cayenne pepper, (optional)
- 1 tbsp nutritional yeast flakes
- 1 tsp sea salt, omit if using vegetable bouillons
- 1 bay leaf

INSTRUCTIONS

1. Heat the oil in a large pot on medium high heat.

2. Add onion and cook until soft, or for about 4 minutes.

3. Add garlic, celery, green onions and cook for 2 minutes, stirring constantly.

4. Stir in carrots, thyme, parsley, basil, and cabbage.

5. Cook for another 2 minutes. Add water or broth, bay leaf, yeast flakes, paprika, cayenne pepper and salt.

6. Cover pot and bring to a boil. Reduce the heat to simmer for 20-30 minutes.

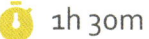 1h 30m 8

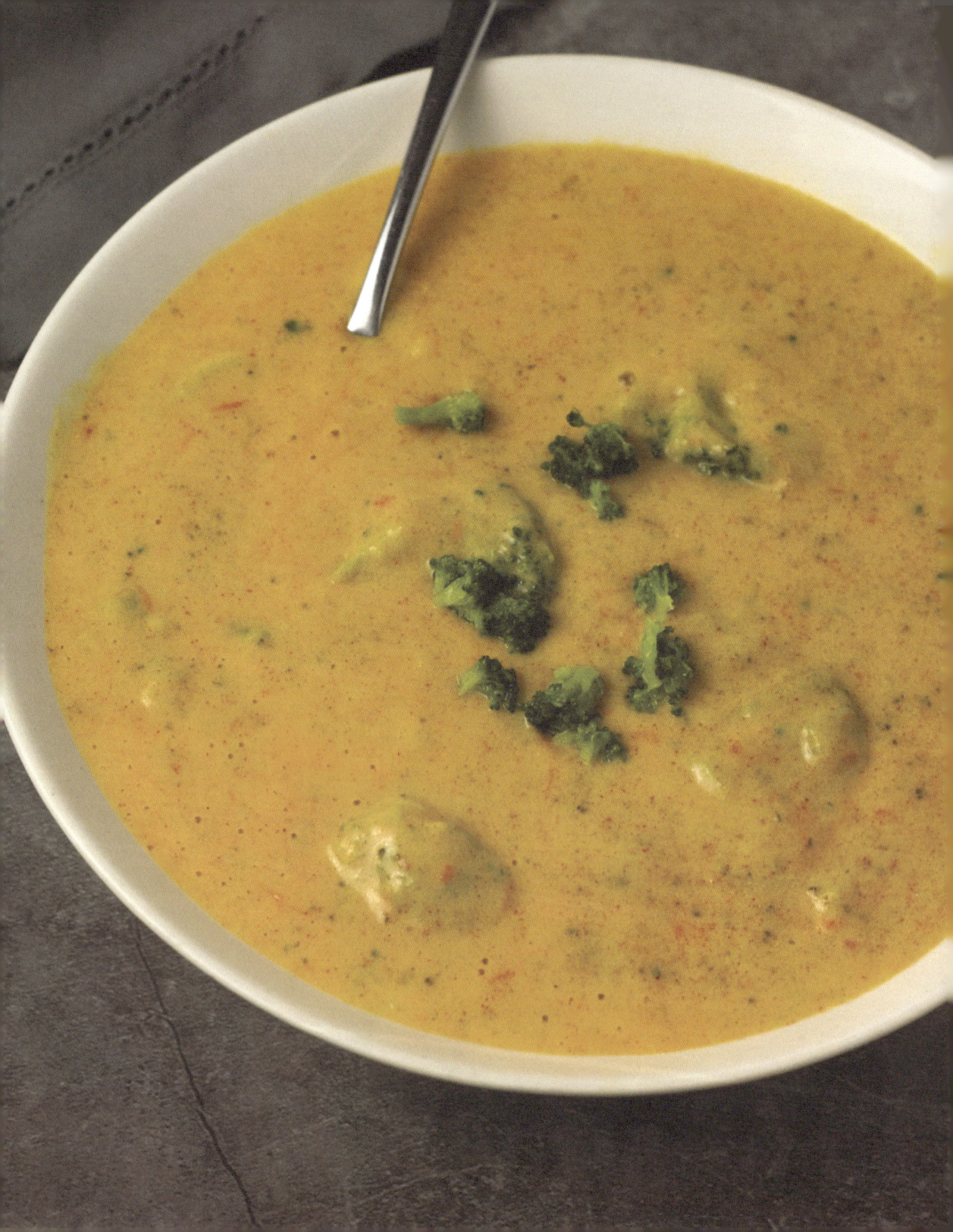

BROCCOLI CHEESE SOUP

Flavorful, creamy and comforting vegan broccoli cheese soup is packed with lots of fiber and nutrients from broccoli and sweet potatoes!

INGREDIENTS

- 4 cups broccoli florets, chopped
- 1 tablespoon olive oil, or 1/4 cup vegetable broth for sauteing
- 1 medium onion, chopped
- 2 cloves garlic, minced
- 3 cups vegetable broth
- 1 cup water
- 1/2 cup raw cashews, soaked for 1 hour
- 1/2 cup cooked sweet potatoes
- 3 tablespoons nutritional yeast flakes
- 1 tablespoon onion, chopped
- 1 clove garlic
- 1 teaspoon salt
- 1/4 teaspoon Cayenne pepper

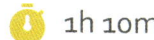 1h 10m   4

INSTRUCTIONS

1. Heat a large saucepan with oil or water over medium-high heat.

2. Add onion and saute until soft, or for about 4 minutes.

3. Stir in garlic and cook for 1 minute. Add broccoli florets stir to coat, add vegetable broth and bring to boil.

4. Reduce heat to simmer for 5 minutes or until broccoli is tender. Meanwhile, prepare the cheese sauce.

CHEESE SAUCE

1. Place cashews and water in a blender and process until smooth. Add sweet potatoes, yeast flakes onion, garlic, salt, and pepper and continue processing until smooth and creamy.

2. Transfer cheese sauce into a bowl and set aside.

3. Take half the broccoli soup and pulse in a blender (I prefer it to be chunky).

4. Return the blended soup to the saucepan along with the cheesy sauce and cook stirring until thickened.

5. Enjoy on its own or baked potato, or bread.

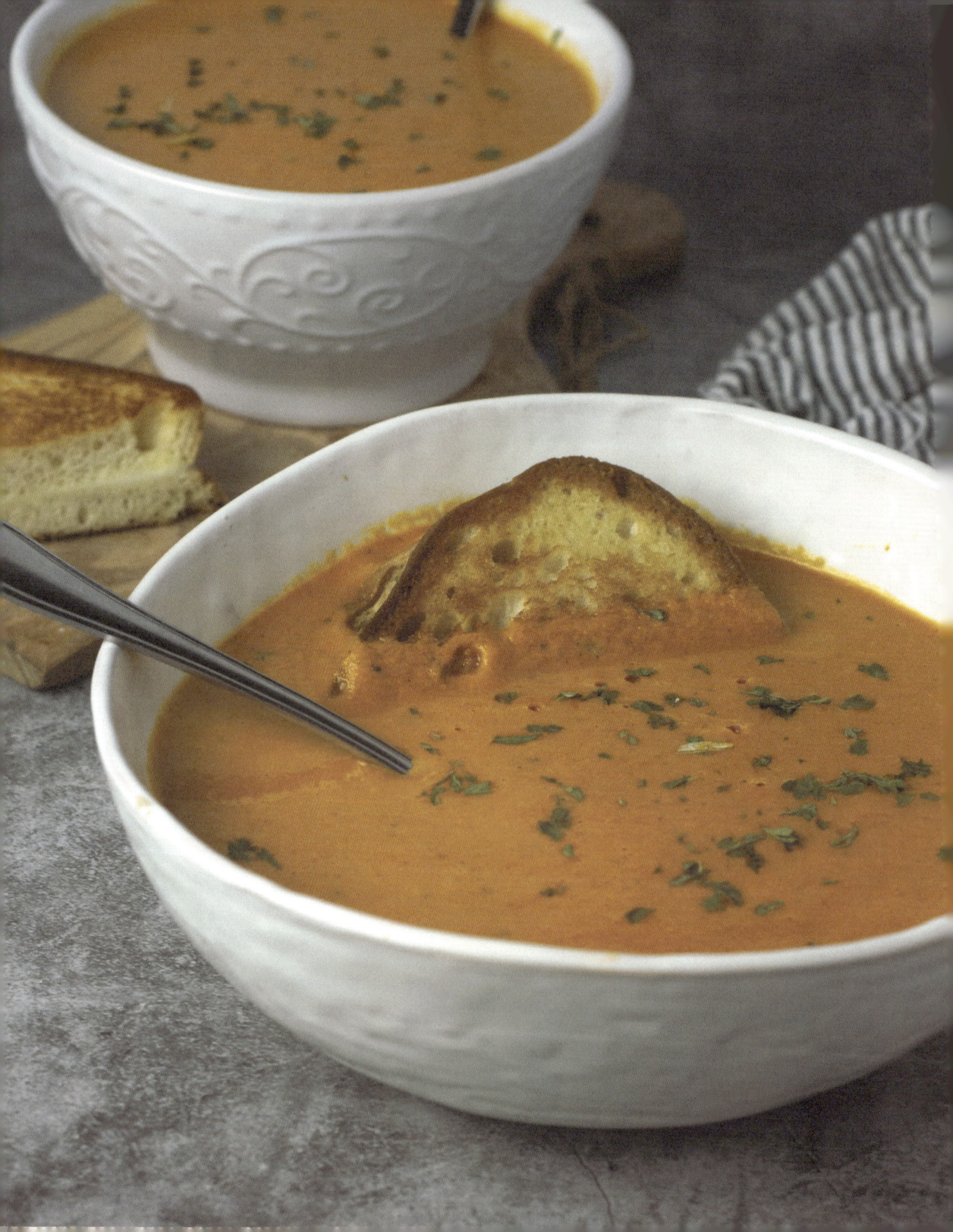

TOMATO SOUP

This vegan tomato soup recipe is so easy to prepare, and is rich and creamy. The perfect comfort soup that tastes amazingly fresh, with incredibly flavorful classic tomato soup flavor!

INGREDIENTS

- 1 1/2 cups water
- 1/2 cup raw cashews
- 2 tablespoons extra-virgin olive oil
- 1 small yellow onion, quartered
- 3 cloves garlic, quartered
- 1 28 oz can tomatoes, whole peeled (liquid included)
- 3 cups vegetable broth
- 2 teaspoons basil, dried or 2 tablespoons fresh
- 2 teaspoons dried oregano
- 1 teaspoon dried thyme
- 2 teaspoons cane sugar
- salt, to taste

INSTRUCTIONS

1. Add water and cashews to a blender, and process until smooth.

2. In a large pot, heat olive oil on medium-low heat. Sauté onion and garlic for about 2 minutes. Add blended cashew mixture, canned tomato, vegetable broth, dried herbs, and sugar.

3. Bring to a boil on medium-high heat, then reduce to the lowest setting and let simmer for 10 minutes.

4. Add salt to taste (I used one tablespoon for reference). Blend in batches until smooth, then serve while hot.

5. You can also let this cool at room temperature, then keep in your fridge for up to 5 days, reheating small amounts as necessary.

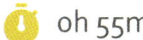 oh 55m   4

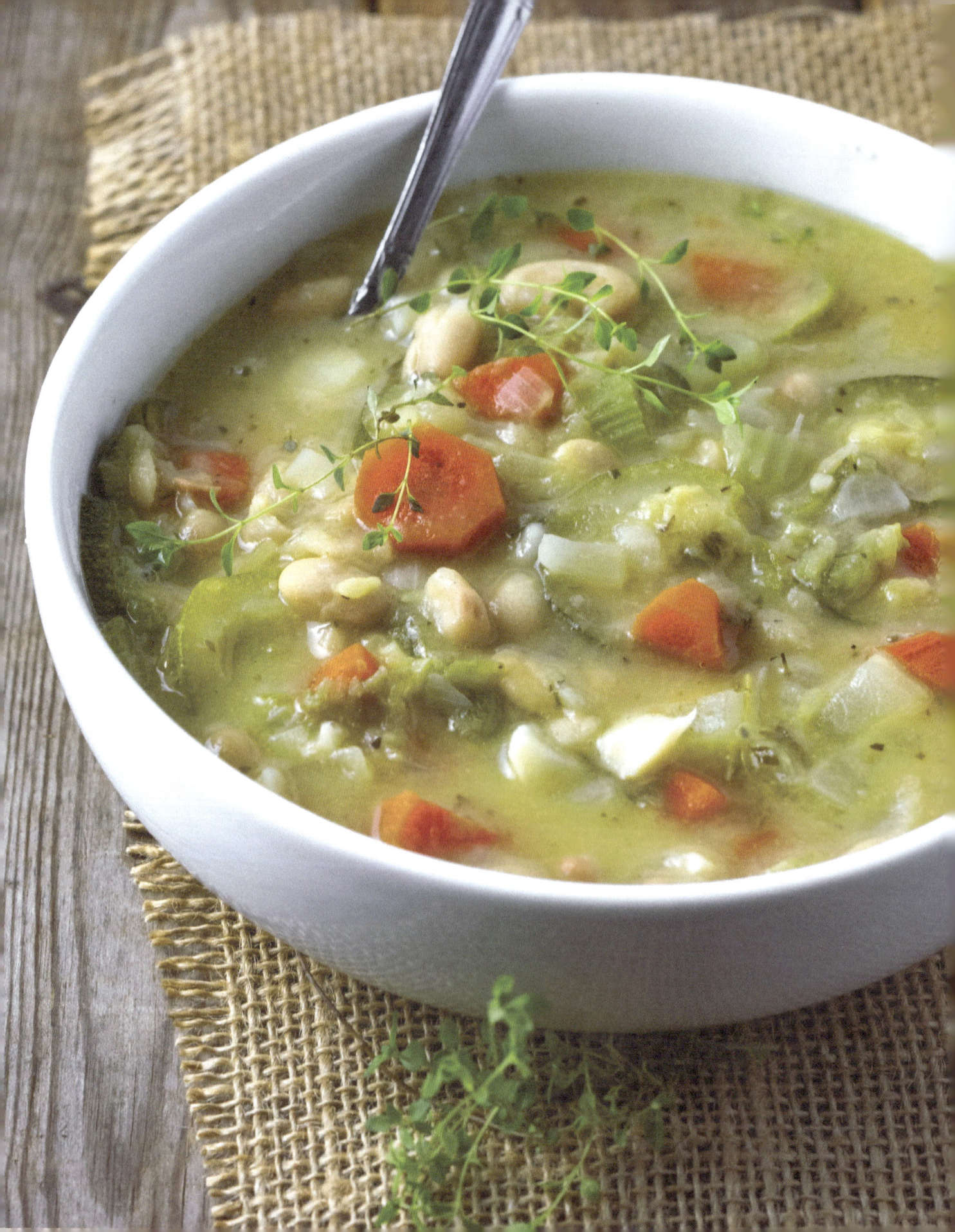

ZUCCHINI SOUP

This vegan zucchini soup is bursting with flavor, freshly grown zucchini, white bean, onion, garlic, and herbs. A healthy creamy zucchini soup that is vegan and gluten-free.

INGREDIENTS

- 1 tablespoon olive oil
- 1 small onion, finely chopped
- 3 cloves garlic, minced
- 1 green onion, chopped
- 1 celery stalk, chopped
- 1 sprig fresh thyme, or ¼ teaspoon dried thyme
- ½ teaspoon Italian seasoning
- 2 medium zucchini, cut into slices
- 1 medium carrot, diced
- 1 (15 ounce) can white beans
- 3 cups vegetable broth
- ¼ teaspoon cayenne pepper, or to taste
- salt, to taste

INSTRUCTIONS

1. Heat oil in a pot on medium-high heat. Add onion, garlic, green onion, celery, thyme, Italian seasoning and cook until onion is soft.

2. Add zucchini, carrots, white beans (optional to rinse and drain beans), vegetable broth, cayenne pepper and salt to taste.

3. Bring soup to boil, reduce heat to simmer for about 20 minutes, until thick.

4. You can add extra vegetable broth if your soup is too thick, if your soup is too thin, cook for longer. Mash some of the beans with a fork and it will help to thicken the soup as well.

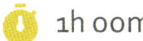 1h 00m 8

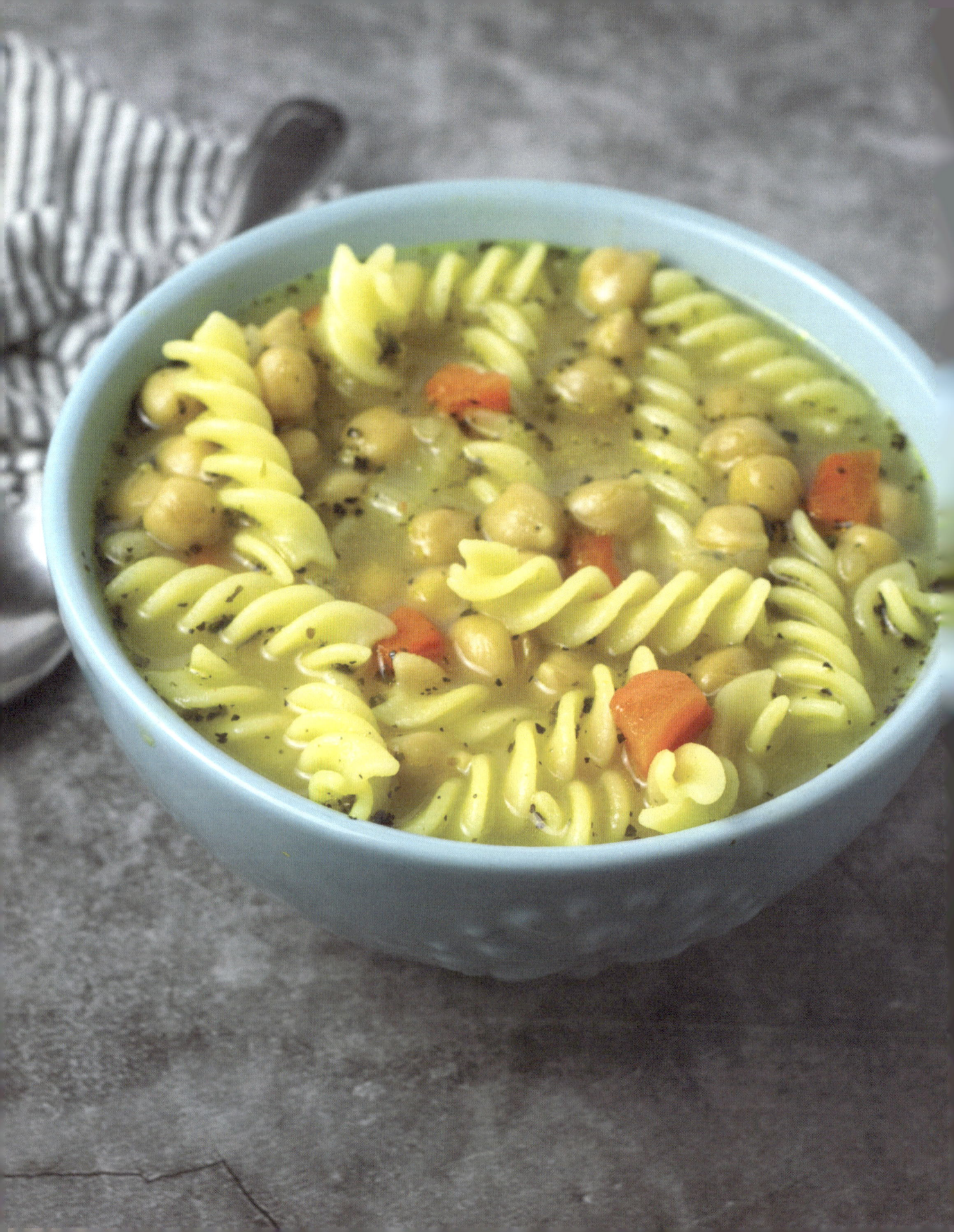

CHICKPEA NOODLE SOUP

Here is a delicious vegan chicken noodle soup is the ultimate comfort dish, it is so hearty and perfect to fight off a cold especially during the colder months.

INGREDIENTS

- 1 tablespoon olive oil
- 1 large onion, diced
- 4 cloves garlic, minced
- 3 stalks celery, chopped
- 2 carrots, chopped
- 2 sprigs fresh thyme
- 1 teaspoon ground coriander
- 1 teaspoon Italian seasoning
- ¼ teaspoon ground turmeric
- 1 teaspoon nutritional yeast flakes
- 1 (14 ounce) can chickpeas, drained
- 5 cups vegetable broth
- ¼ cup coconut milk
- 4 ounces gluten-free pasta of choice
- 2 tablespoons fresh parsley, chopped

INSTRUCTIONS

1. Heat oil in large pot on medium-high heat. Add onion and cook until soft, or for about 3 minutes.

2. Stir in garlic, celery, carrots, thyme, coriander, Italian seasoning, ground turmeric, yeast flakes and cook stirring for 3 minutes.

3. Add chickpeas, water/broth, coconut milk and bring to a boil.

4. Stir in pasta and simmer for about 10-15 minutes or until pasta is cooked. My need to add an extra cup of water.

5. Stir in parsley and salt. Delicious served with salad.

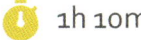 1h 10m 6

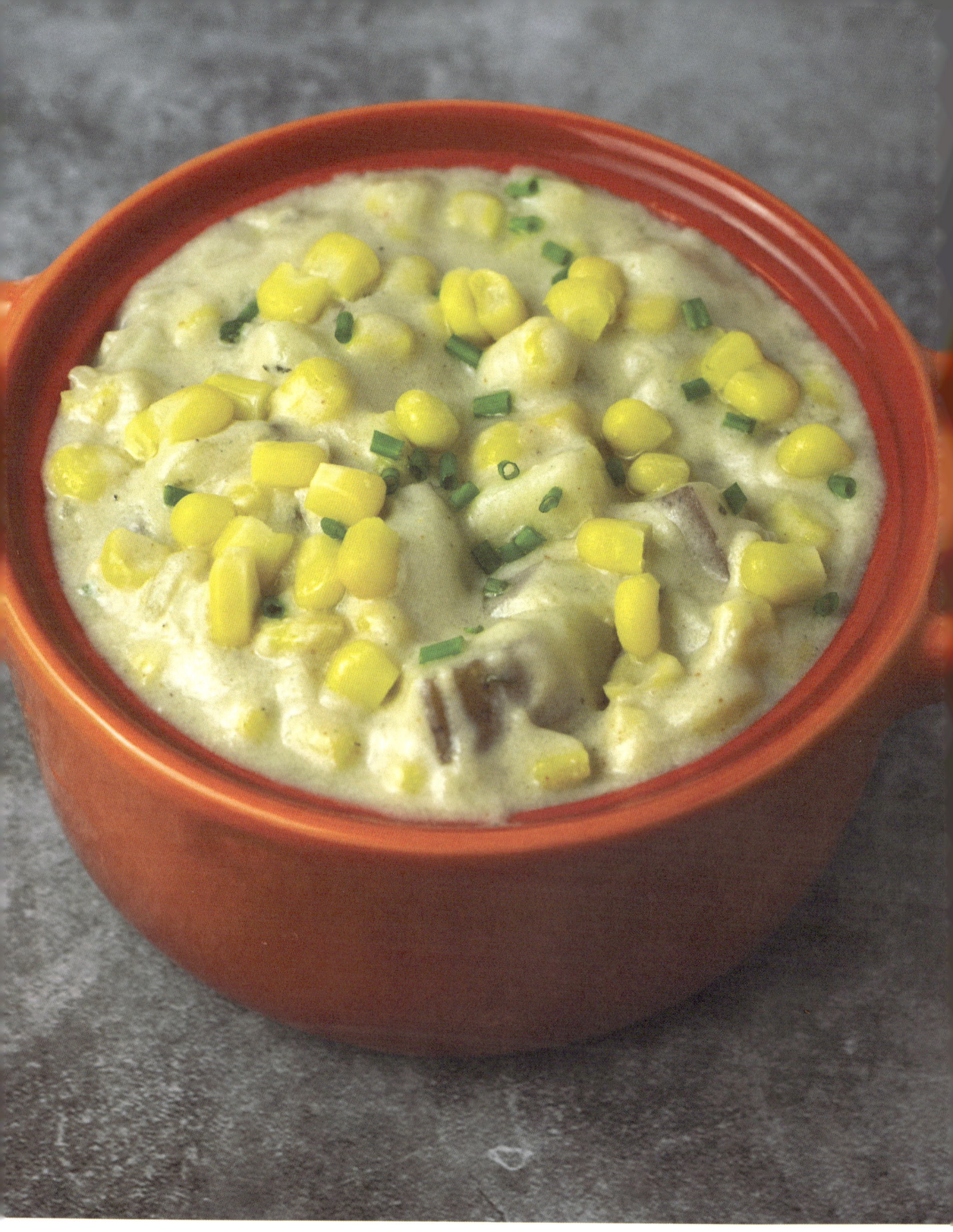

CORN CHOWDER

This creamy, sweet, delicious soup is perfect for your family and entertaining. Using a roux made with vegan butter and gluten free flour and a cashew cream as thickening, means this soup is creamy and luscious as it gets.

INGREDIENTS

- 1 tablespoon olive oil
- 1 large onion, diced
- 4 cloves garlic, minced
- 3 stalks celery, chopped
- 2 carrots, chopped
- 2 sprigs fresh thyme
- 1 teaspoon ground coriander
- 1 teaspoon Italian seasoning
- ¼ teaspoon ground turmeric
- 1 teaspoon nutritional yeast flakes
- 1 (14 ounce) can chickpeas, drained
- 5 cups vegetable broth
- ¼ cup coconut milk
- 4 ounces gluten-free pasta of choice
- 2 tablespoons fresh parsley, chopped

INSTRUCTIONS

1. Melt butter in a large pot over medium heat. Add onions and sauté until soft, about three minutes. Add garlic after about a minute, then add flour while stirring.

2. In a blender, process milk and cashews until completely smooth. Add cashew cream, broth, and water to pot. Add corn, potatoes, yeast flakes, thyme, and paprika.

3. Bring to boil, then lower heat, cover, and simmer for 30 minutes, adding broth if the soup thickens too much. Blend half, or partially using an immersion blender. Add salt to taste, and garnish with chives.

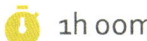 1h 00m   4

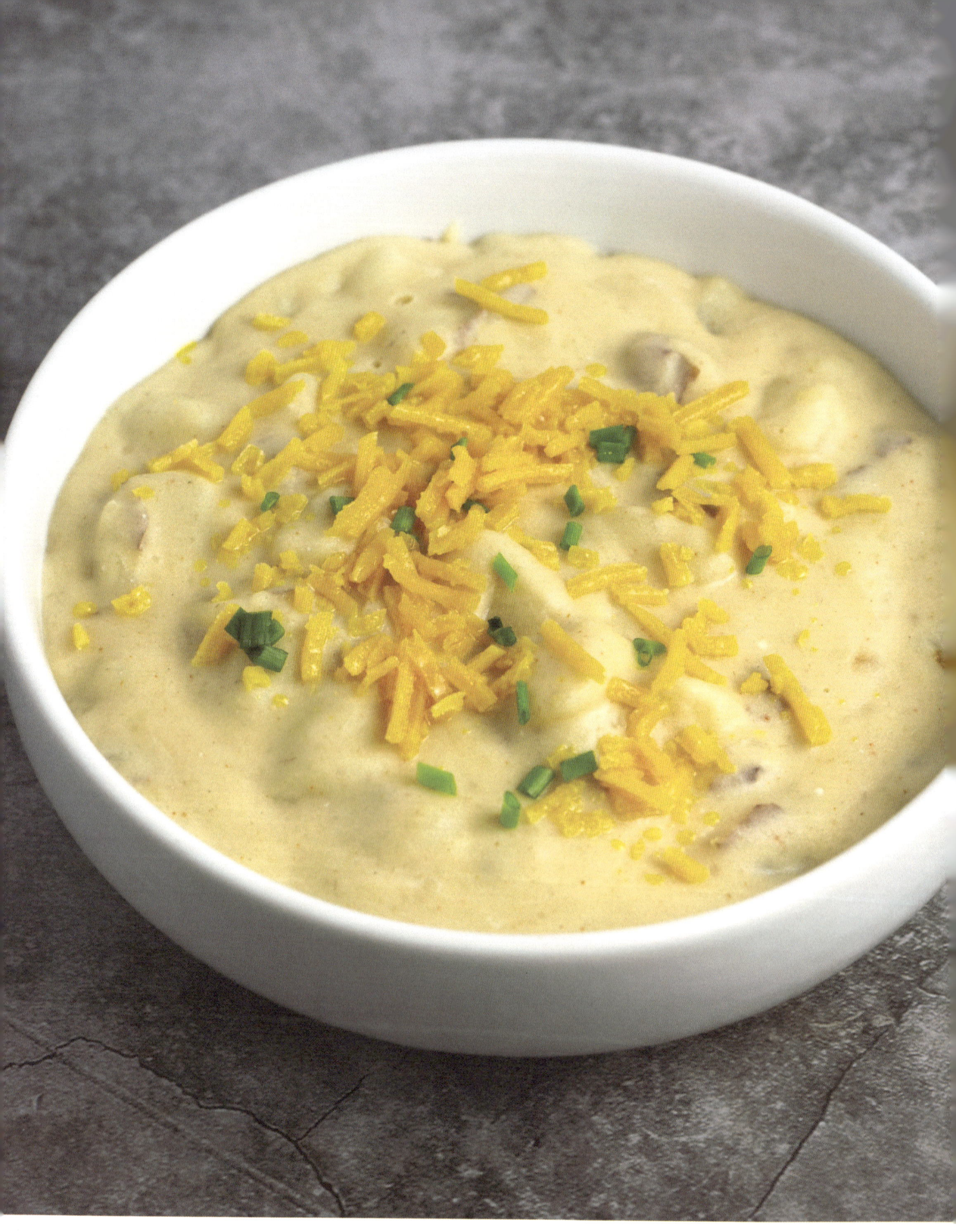

CREAMY POTATO SOUP

This soup is one of those classics, and for very good reasons. There is not much that this soup won't fix, or at least help you feel better. Cooked potatoes are very creamy, especially when blended with milk, making this soup just as creamy as it would be with cream.

INGREDIENTS

- ¼ cup butter
- ¼ cup gluten free all-purpose flour
- 2 cups onion, diced
- 4 cloves of garlic, diced
- 4 cups broth
- 2 cups unsweetened non-dairy milk
- 6 cups potatoes, diced
- 2 celery stalks, diced
- 1 carrot, diced
- ¼ cup vegan bacon, chopped (optional)
- 2 tablespoons nutritional yeast flakes
- 2 teaspoons smoked paprika
- 1 teaspoon Dijon mustard
- salt, to taste
- Garnishing ideas
    - Sour cream
    - Chopped chives
    - Green onions
    - Vegan bacon pieces

INSTRUCTIONS

1. Melt butter over medium heat in a large pot. Add onions and sauté for three minutes, then add garlic and sauté for one minute.

2. Add flour while stirring, then add broth, milk, potatoes, celery, carrots, vegan bacon, yeast flakes, paprika, and mustard. Bring to boil then cover and simmer on low for 30 minutes.

3. Blend some or all of the soup, depending on your preference, for a creamy texture.

4. Garnish with the ingredients of your choice.

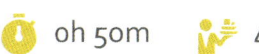 0h 50m   4

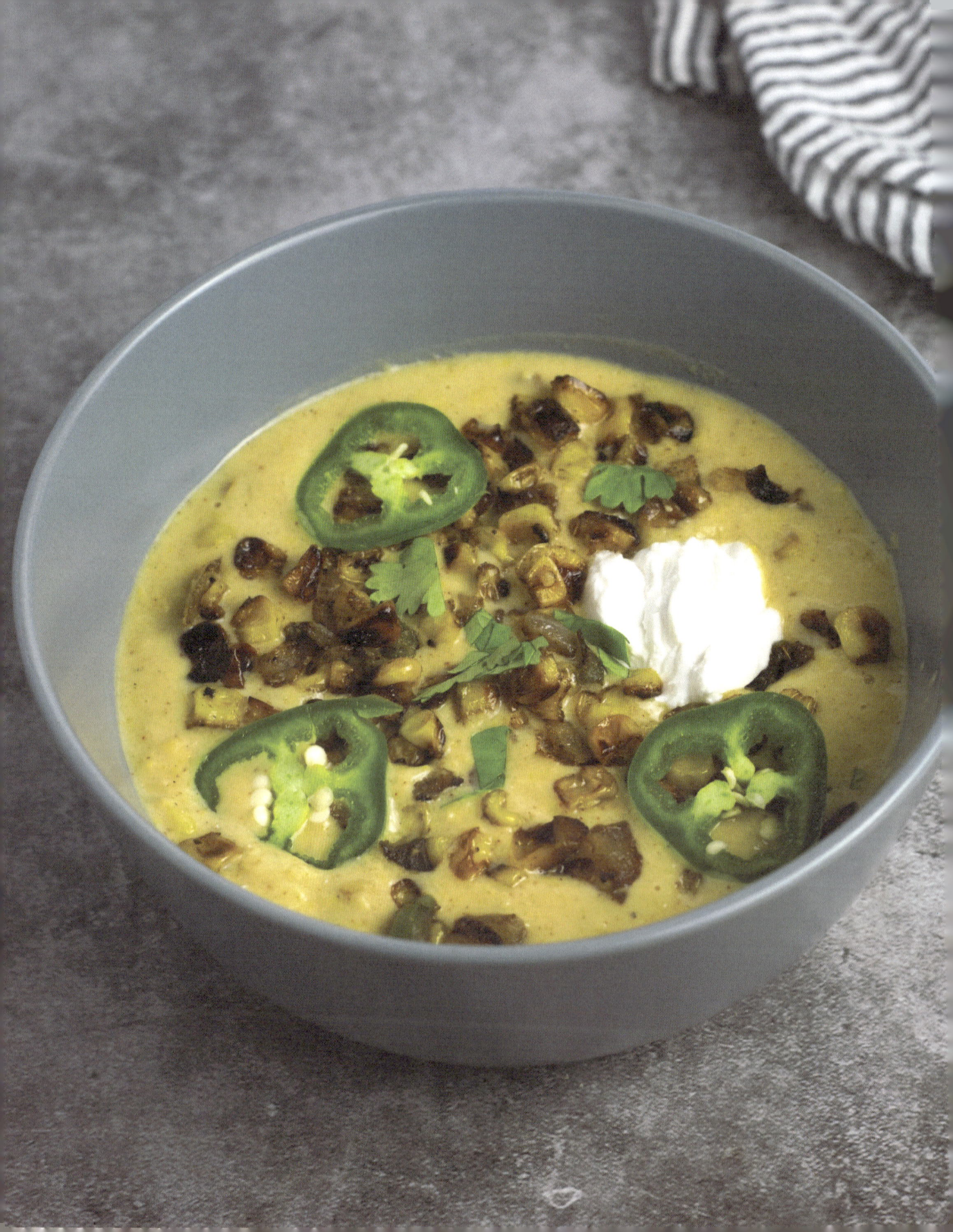

MEXICAN STREET CORN SOUP

I love Mexican street corn. It is such a great side or snack. Putting it into soup form is a genius move, and it tastes so good. Adding a bit of chipotle chili powder, which is made from smoked chili peppers, adds a bit of smokiness that takes this soup up to the next level.

INGREDIENTS

- 1 tablespoon butter
- 1 cup corn
- ½ cup onions, diced
- 1 jalapeño, diced
- 2 teaspoons cumin powder
- 1 teaspoon chipotle chili powder
- 1 tablespoon butter
- ½ cup onions, diced
- 1 red bell pepper, diced
- 2 cloves garlic, minced
- 4 cups corn
- 4 cups vegetable broth
- 1 cup unsweetened non-dairy milk
- ½ cup sour cream
- ½ lime, juiced
- salt, to taste
- **Garnishing ideas**
  - charred corn
  - cilantro

INSTRUCTIONS

1. In a small frying pan, melt the butter on medium heat. Add onion and sauté until soft, then and corn, jalapeno, and garlic. Continue until corn is blackened in spots, then add cumin and chipotle powder. Stir for a minute then set aside.

2. In a large pot, sauté onion on medium-low heat until soft, about 2 minutes. Add red bell pepper and garlic for another minute. Add corn, broth, and milk. Cover and simmer for 20 minutes.

3. Use an immersion blender and process lightly, or blend half in a blender. Add sour cream, lime, and salt to taste.

4. Garnish with ingredients of choice.

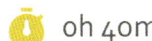 0h 40m   6

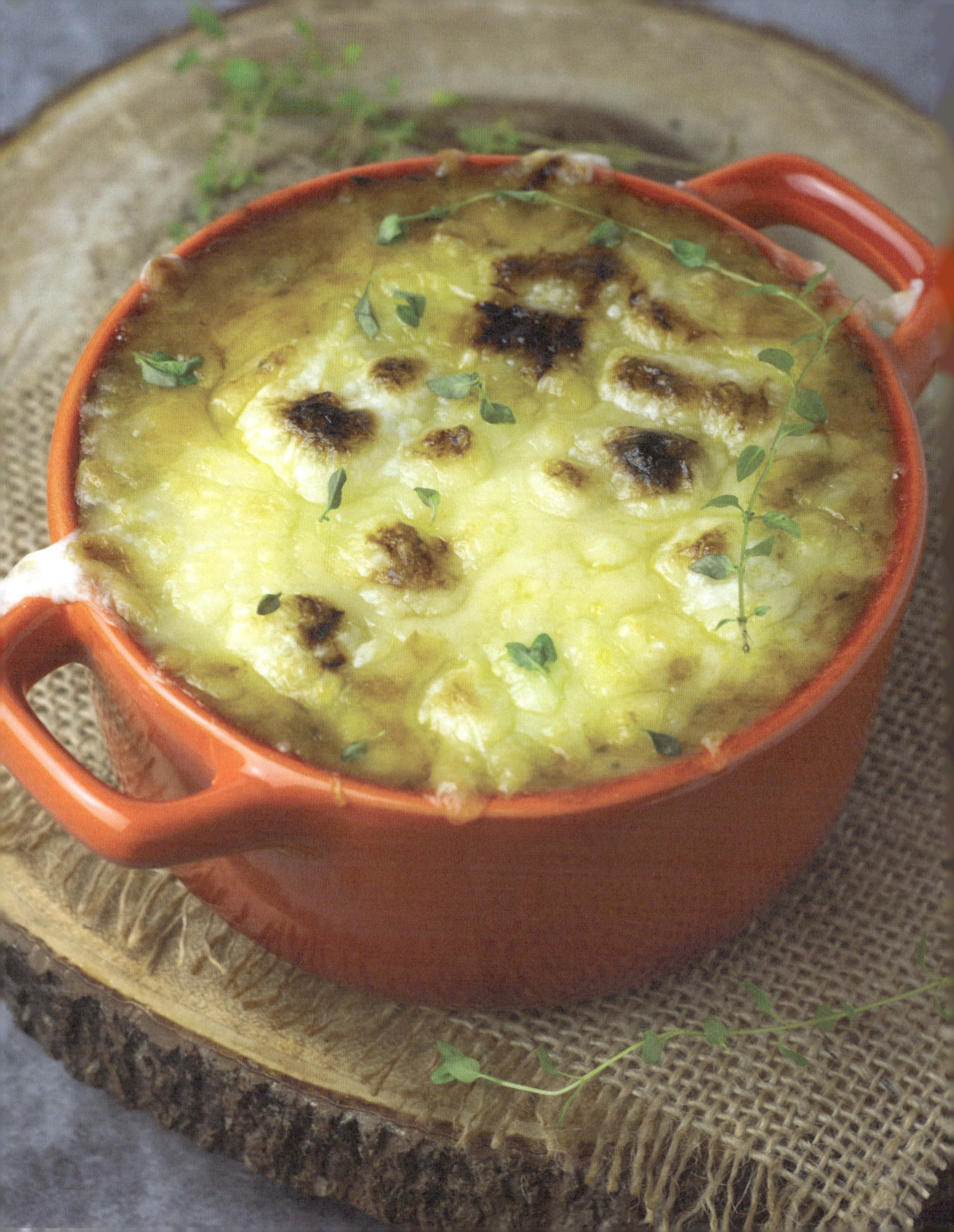

FRENCH ONION SOUP

Yummy caramelized onion goodness, perfect with melted stretchy vegan cheese and a crusty buttered baguette. I mean, it's a classic. Also, surprisingly simple to make. What else could I possibly say?

INGREDIENTS

- 3 tablespoons vegan butter
- 6 large yellow onions, chopped
- 1 cup vegetable broth (optional)
- 4 cloves garlic, minced
- 6 cups broth
- 1 teaspoon Worcestershire sauce
- 1 teaspoon thyme
- bay leaf
- vegan mozzarella, for topping

INSTRUCTIONS

1. Melt butter in a large pot on medium heat. Add onions, and turn down to low after 3 minutes. Leave on low, stirring occasionally until dark brown, usually for 30-40 minutes. Add vegetable broth if the onions become too dry and start to stick.

2. Add garlic and continue to stir occasionally for two minutes. Add broth, Worcestershire sauce, thyme, and bay leaf. Cover and simmer for 20 minutes.

3. Remove bay leaf. When serving, top with vegan mozzarella shreds.

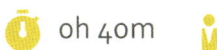 0h 40m   4

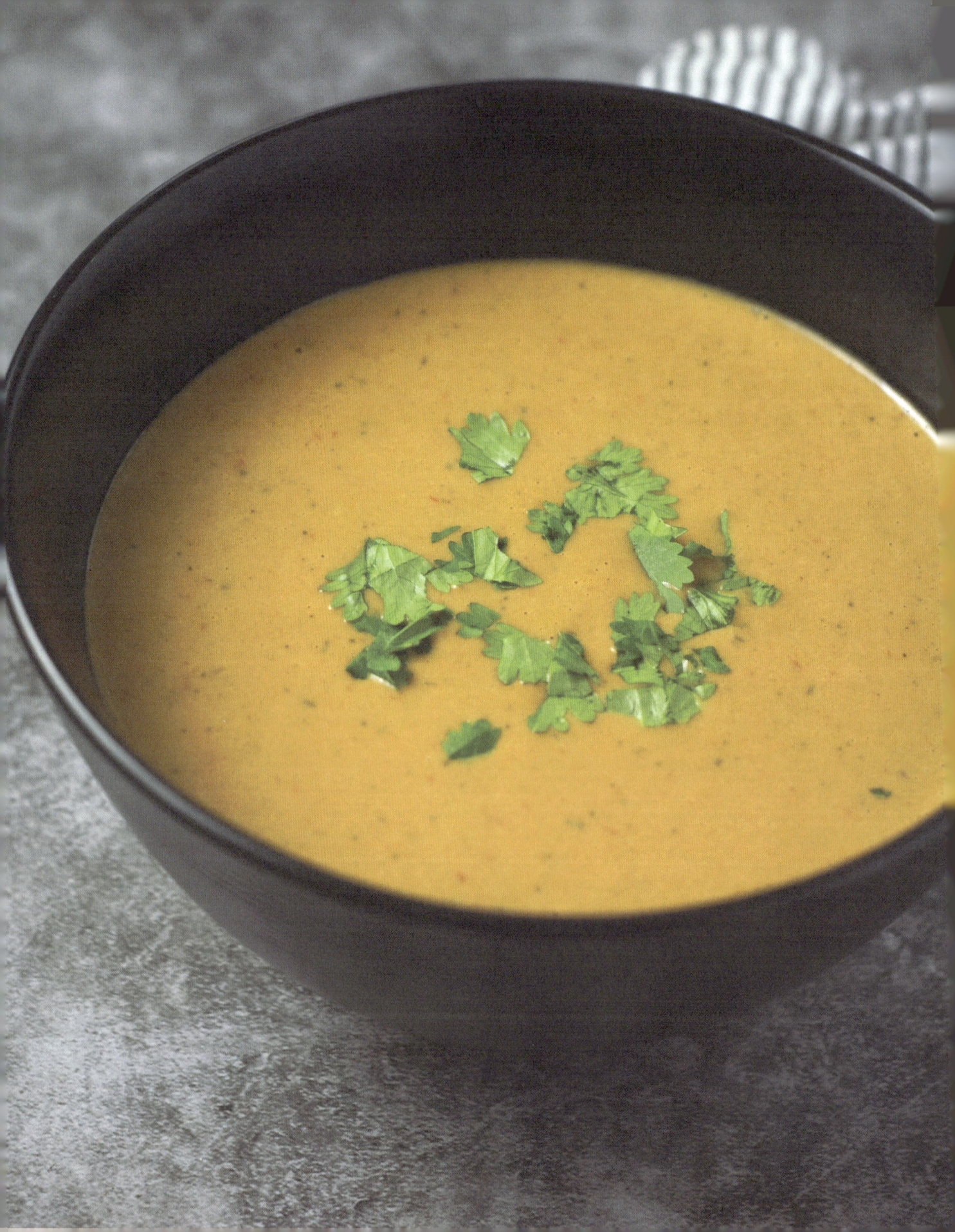

ROASTED RED PEPPER SOUP

I love the wonderful flavor of roasted red peppers, and it's the sort of lovely savory flavor that makes a perfect soup. Roast the garlic as well for extra roasted goodness!

INGREDIENTS

- 6 red bell peppers
- 6 cloves garlic
- 2 tablespoons olive oil
- 2 cups onion, diced
- 3 pieces of sundried tomatoes, minced
- 2 cups water
- 1 ½ cups cashews
- 1 cup vegetable broth
- 2 teaspoons thyme
- 2 teaspoons oregano
- 1 teaspoon sriracha (optional)
- bay leaf

INSTRUCTIONS

1. Preheat oven to 400° F. Slice red bell peppers in half, then scoop out the seeds and white fleshy bits. Place the bell peppers skin up on a lined baking sheet. Bake until the skins are charred and wrinkled, about 20-25 minutes.

2. Place the peppers into a sealed plastic container or zipper bag, to use the heat and steam to loosen the skin of the peppers. Allow them to cool, then peel off any burnt skin.

3. In a large pot, heat oil on medium heat. Sauté onions for two minutes, then add garlic, sun-dried tomatoes, and peppers for another minute.

4. While sautéing the vegetables, blend the water and cashews until smooth. Add the cashew cream, water, herbs, and optional sriracha if you want a little kick.

5. Cover and simmer for 15 minutes, remove bay leaf, then blend in batches or with immersion blender. Add salt as needed.

 0h 40m 4

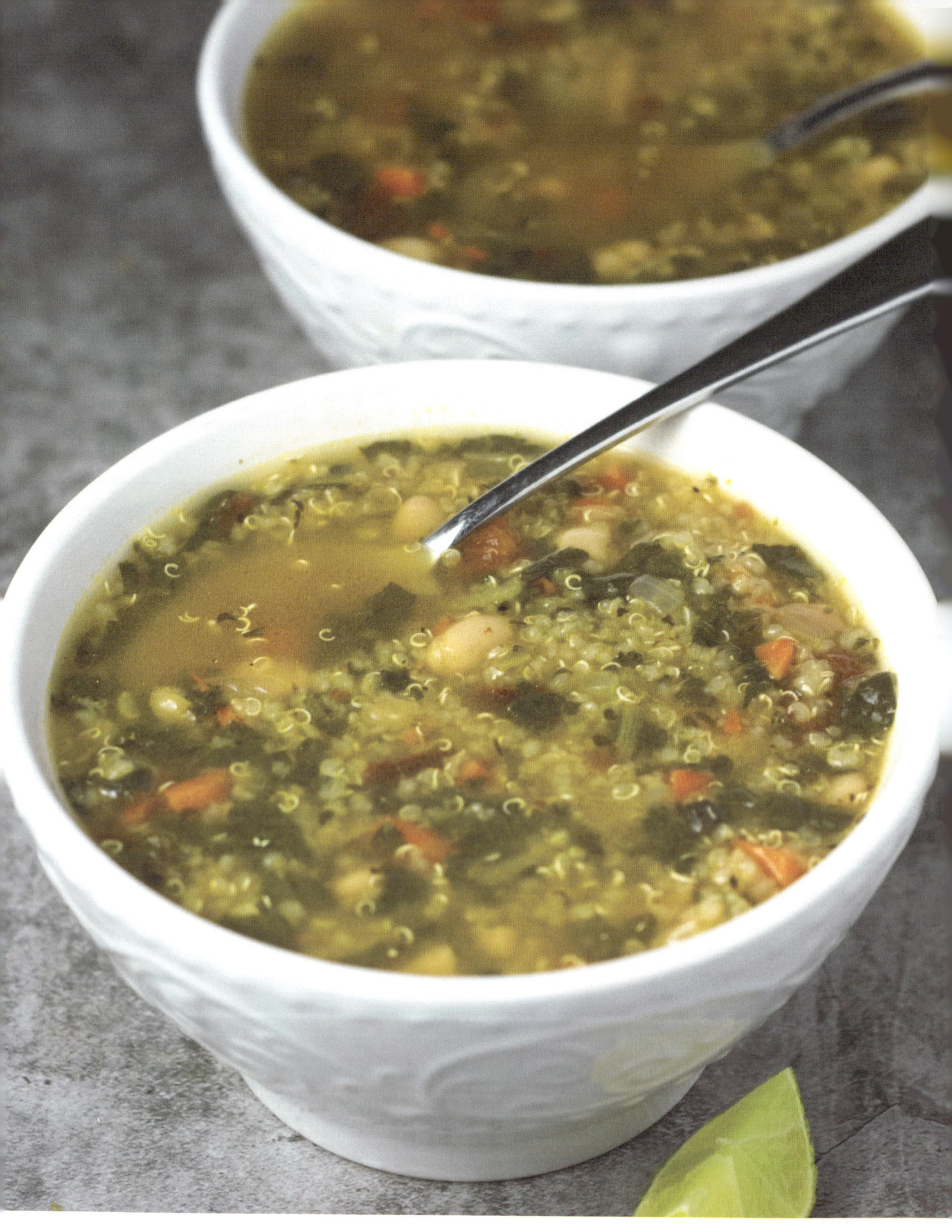

QUINOA VEGETABLE SOUP

This soup is a comforting warm broth based vegetable soup, but with the addition of quinoa, becomes a hearty dish that can be a wonderful dinner with some crusty bread. It is already filled with quinoa, carrots, chickpeas, spinach, and more, but you can feel free to add or substitute your favorites.

INGREDIENTS

- 1 tablespoon olive oil
- 2 cups onion, diced
- 4-6 cloves garlic, minced
- 4 celery stalks, diced
- 4 carrots, diced
- 2 cans chickpeas
- 2 cups quinoa, rinsed
- 2 cups spinach, frozen
- 6 sun-dried tomatoes, diced
- 6 cups vegetable broth
- 4 cups water
- 2 tablespoons lemon juice
- 2 teaspoons thyme
- 2 teaspoons rosemary
- 1 bay leaf
- salt, to taste

INSTRUCTIONS

1. In a large pot, sauté onions on medium-low heat for three minutes.

2. Add garlic for one minute, then celery, carrots, chickpeas, quinoa, spinach, sun-dried tomatoes, broth, water, lemon, and herbs.

3. Bring to boil, then cover and simmer on low heat for 25 minutes.

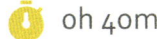 0h 40m   4

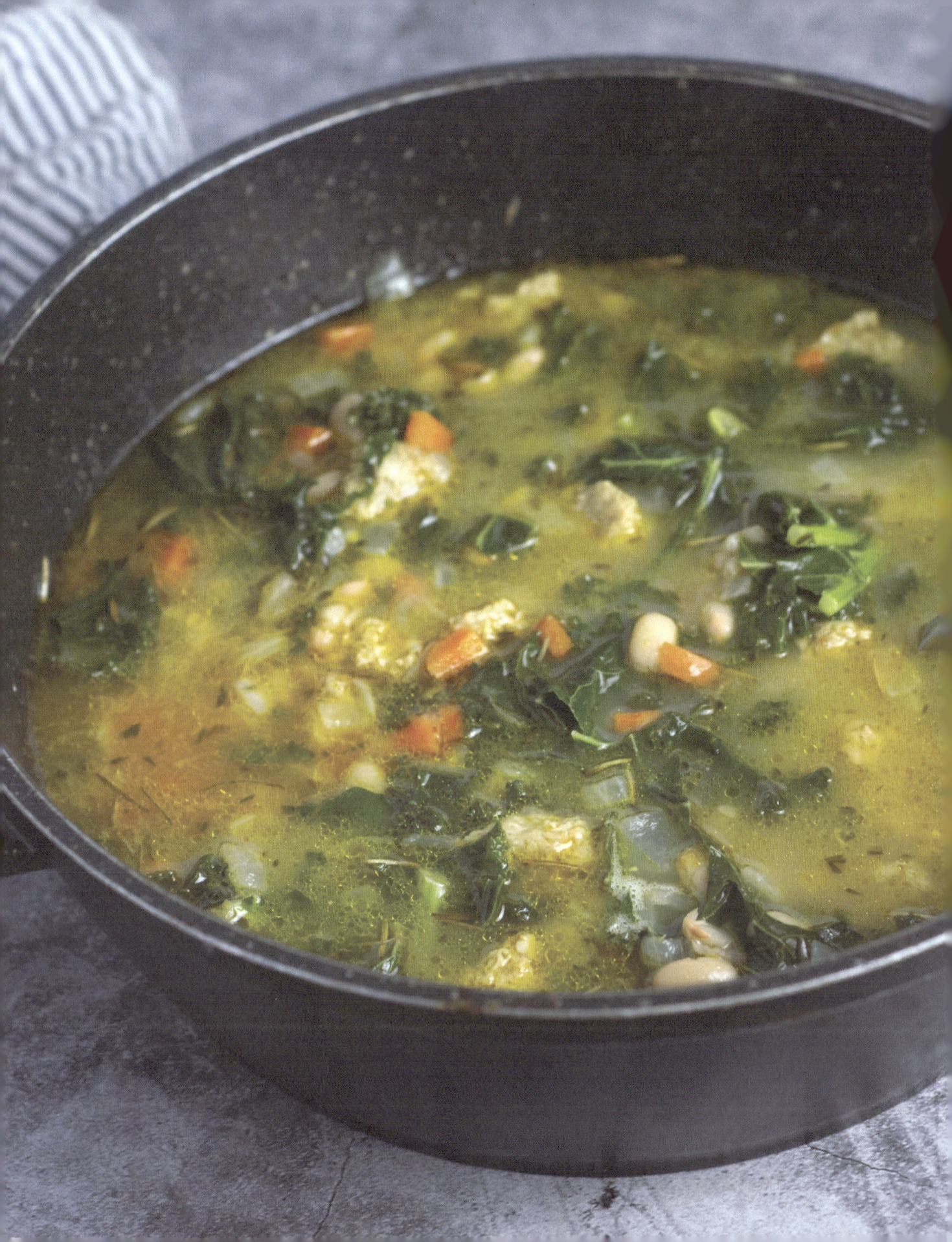

WHITE BEAN & KALE SOUP

This high protein soup can work as a quick hearty lunch, or with dinner. Best of all, it only requires a couple minutes of prep and active cooking, allowing you to go do whatever other important things you have going on.

INGREDIENTS

- 1 tablespoon olive oil
- 2 cups onion
- 6 cloves of garlic
- 2 carrots, diced
- 4 cans white beans
- 6 cups broth
- 4 cups water
- 4 cups kale, chopped
- 2 sausages, broken into chunks
- 2 tablespoon lemon juice
- 1 tablespoon rosemary
- 2 teaspoon thyme
- salt, to taste

INSTRUCTIONS

1. Sauté the onion and garlic in a large pot over medium heat.

2. Add the rest of the ingredients, bring to boil, then simmer for 20 minutes.

3. Add salt as necessary.

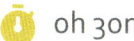 0h 30m   4

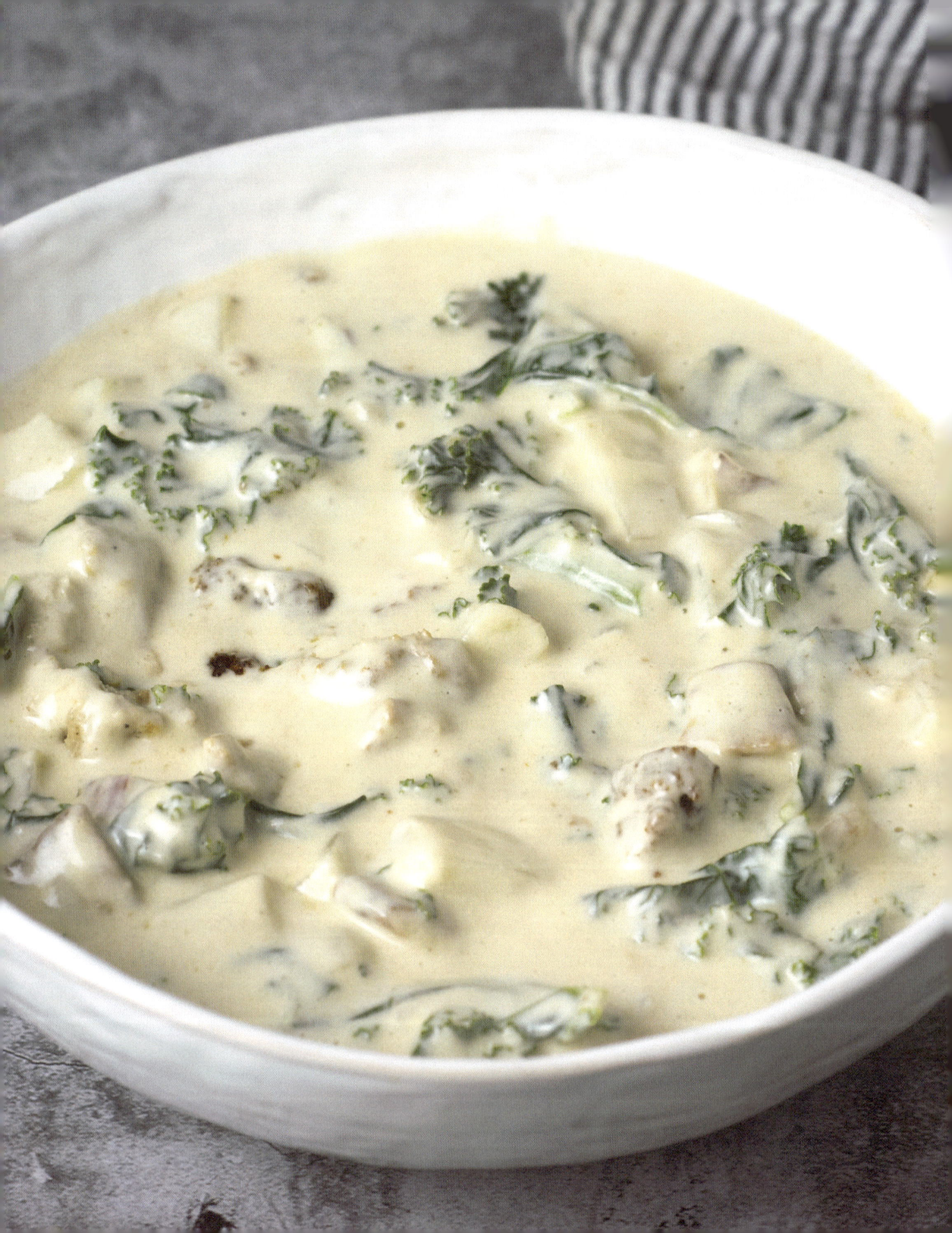

TUSCAN SAUSAGE KALE SOUP

This is modeled after the famous Zuppa Tuscana, which means "Tuscan soup". It is a creamy based soup with kale, potatoes, and vegan bacon and sausages substitutes, which give the soup a lovely flavor that fits perfectly.

INGREDIENTS

- 1 tablespoon butter or olive oil
- 2 cups sausage, big chunks (I used Beyond sausages)
- 1 cup tempeh bacon (optional)
- 1 tablespoon butter or olive oil
- 2 cups onion, diced
- 4 cloves garlic, minced
- 3 cup milk
- 1 ½ cup cashews
- 6 cups vegetable broth
- 6 potatoes, diced
- 4 cups kale, shredded
- salt, to taste

INSTRUCTIONS

1. In a frying pan, heat butter and fry vegan sausage and bacon substitutes of choice, then set aside.

2. Sauté onions in a large pot over medium heat for three minutes. Add garlic for one minute.

3. Meanwhile, blend milk and cashews into a smooth cream.

4. Add vegetable broth, cashew cream, sausage, bacon, potatoes, and kale to pot.

5. Simmer for 20-30 minutes, or until kale and potatoes are shredded.

6. Add salt to taste

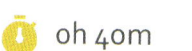 oh 40m   4

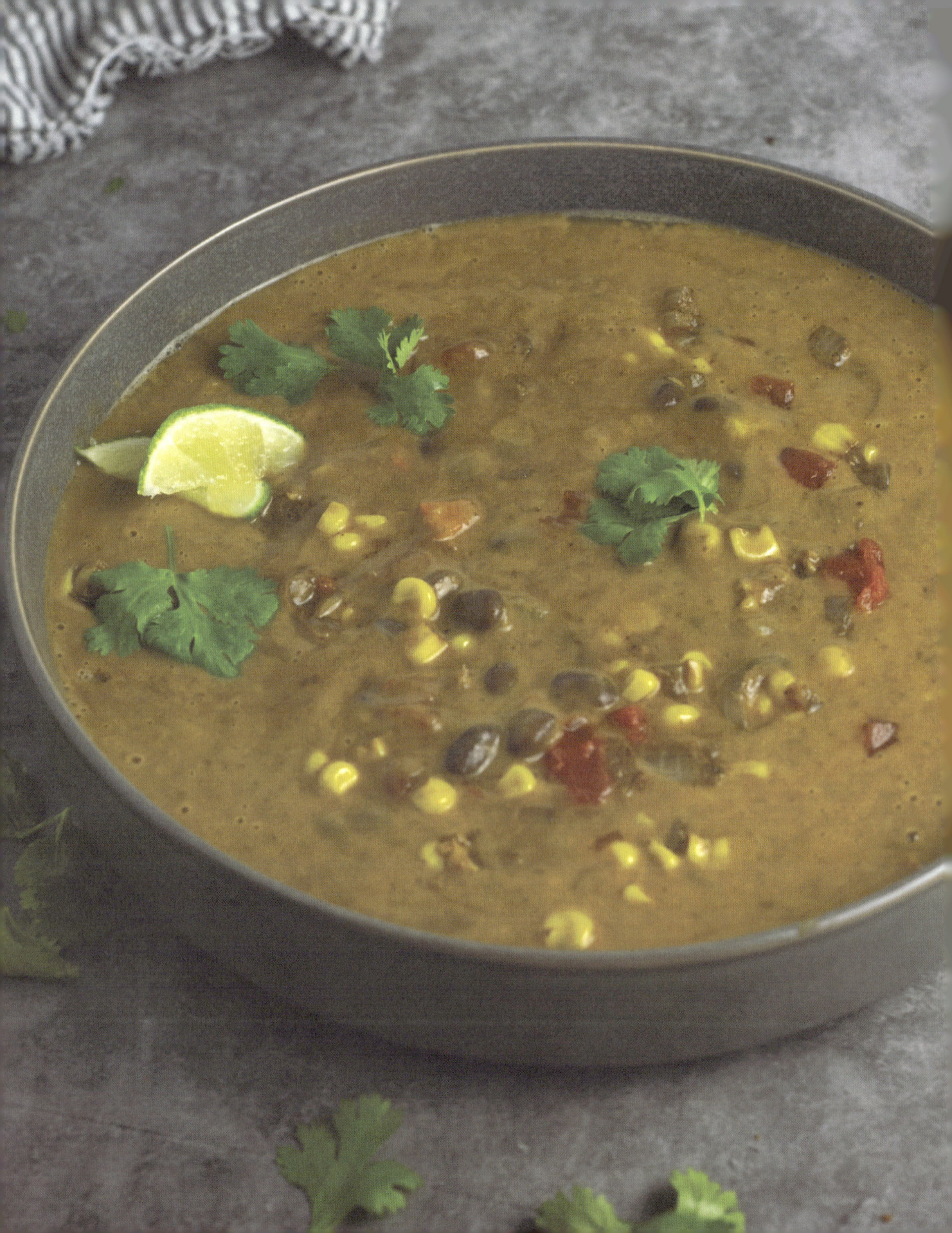

BLACK BEAN SOUP

This healthy hearty soup with southwestern flavors is filled with veggie goodness. It can be a chunky or creamy soup. I do not like to use canned corn for this recipe, so I used frozen; However, you can use fresh.

INGREDIENTS

- 1 tablespoon coconut oil
- 2 cups corn, frozen
- 1 jalapeño, seeded and diced (optional)
- 1 tablespoon cumin
- 1 teaspoon chili powder
- ½ teaspoon chipotle powder (optional)
- 1 tablespoon coconut oil
- ½ onion, diced
- 6-8 garlic cloves, minced
- 1 celery stalk, diced
- 1 carrot, diced
- 2 14 oz. cans diced tomatoes
- 4 15 oz. cans black beans or 4 cups soaked and cooked beans
- 4 cups vegetable broth
- 2 teaspoons lime juice
- salt, to taste
- Garnishing ideas
  - fresh diced tomatoes
  - sour cream
  - cilantro
-

INSTRUCTIONS

1. In a medium-sized pan, heat oil on medium heat. Add corn, jalapeño, and spices, and sauté until corn is browned.

2. In a large pot, heat oil on medium heat. Sauté onions until soft, about three minutes, then add garlic for one minute. Add carrot, celery, tomato, black beans, vegetable broth, and half of the sautéed corn, reserving some as a topping.

3. Simmer on low for 20 minutes, then add lime juice and salt to taste. You can also take out a cup or two and blend for a creamier texture, or use an immersion blender.

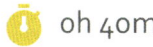 oh 40m   4

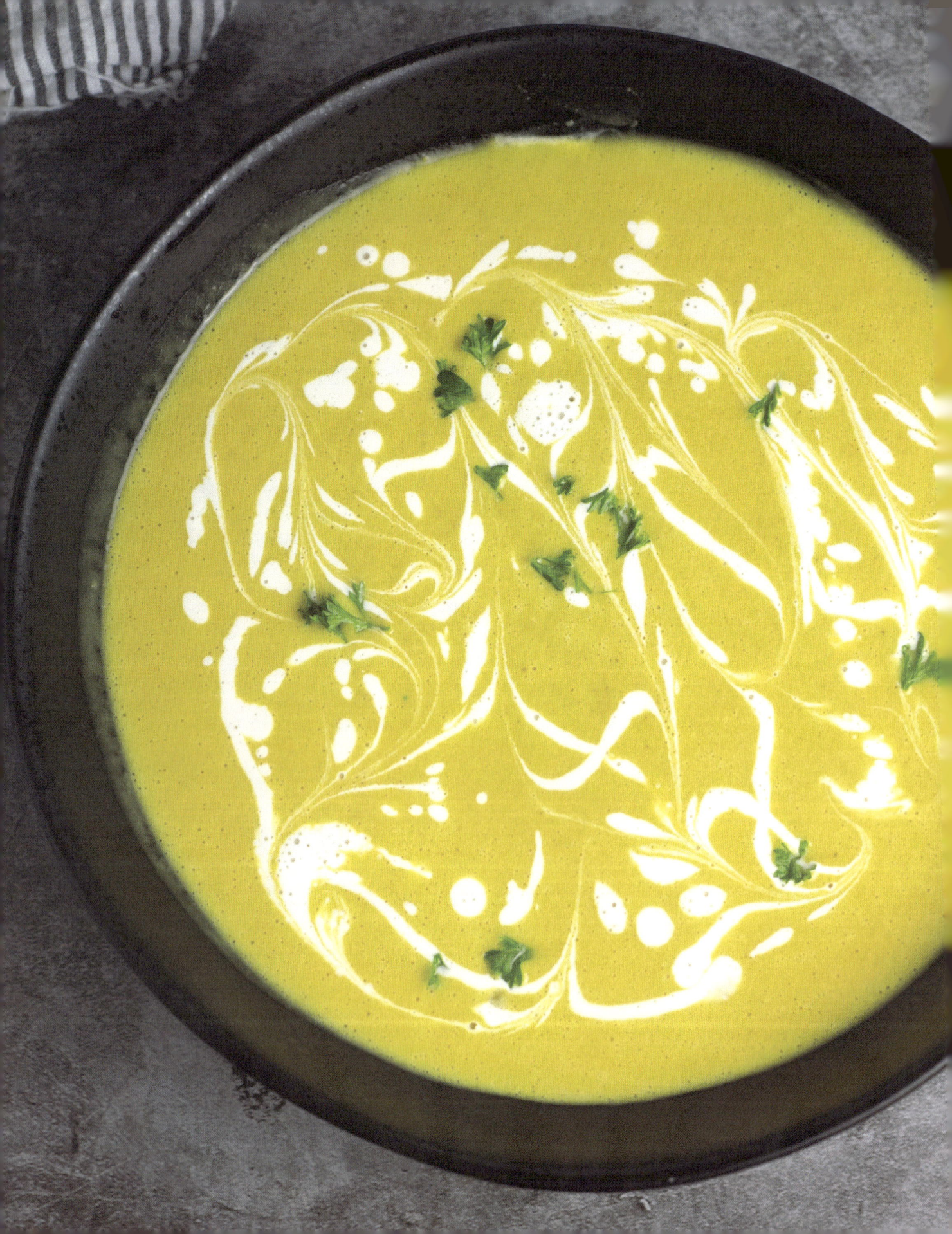

CARROT GINGER SOUP

Roasted carrots make this soup sweet, but yet savory, and the ginger adds a bit of complexity. This is the soup that you entertain with, and have your guests wondering what your secret is. Feel free to add more ginger if you prefer a stronger taste.

INGREDIENTS

- 8 carrots
- 2 tablespoons olive oil
- 1 tsp salt
- Pinch of cayenne (optional)
- 1 tablespoon coconut oil
- 1 cup onion, diced
- 4 cloves garlic, minced
- 3 tablespoons ginger, minced
- ½ teaspoon coriander
- ½ teaspoon cardamom
- ½ teaspoon cumin
- ½ teaspoon allspice
- 6 cups broth
- 3 cups unsweetened non-dairy milk
- 2 cups cashews
- salt, to taste
-

INSTRUCTIONS

1. Preheat oven to 425° F. Place carrots on a lined baking sheet. Drizzle with oil, and rub all over until fully covered, then sprinkle with salt. Roast on top shelf of oven for 40 minutes, turning halfway.

2. Heat oil in a pot on medium-low heat, and sauté onions until soft, for about three minutes. Add garlic and ginger, and continue for another minute. Add roasted carrots, spices, and broth, simmer for 15 minutes.

3. In a blender, process milk and cashews until creamy. Add soup to blender and process until smooth, or add cream to soup and incorporate with hand blender. Add any necessary salt.

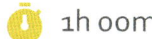 1h 00m   4

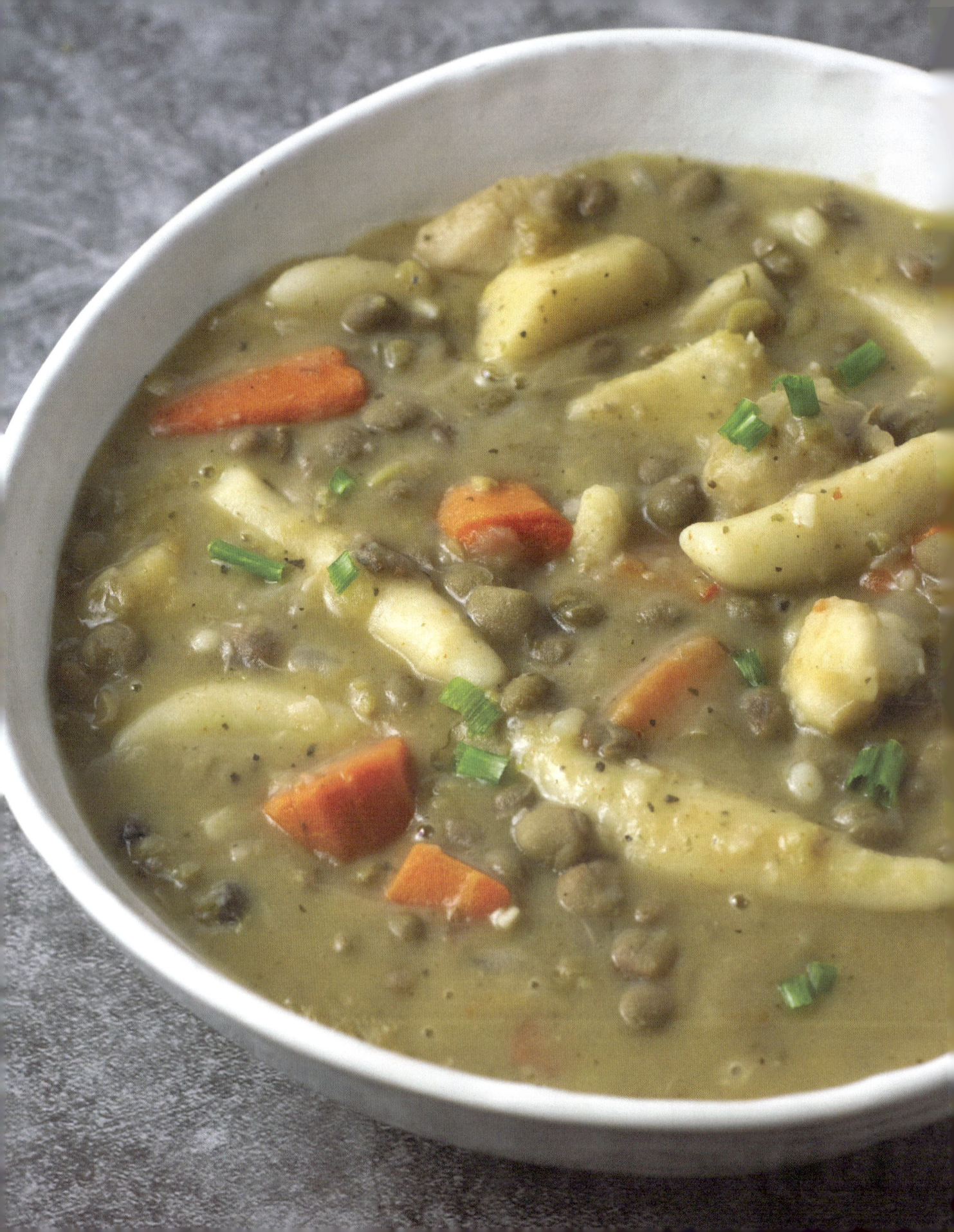

JAMAICAN GUNGO PEAS SOUP

This easy Jamaican gungo peas soup is so delicious and hearty, perfect for the colder months. Full of flavor with gungo peas, yam, carrot, and dumplings.

INGREDIENTS

- 3 cups gungo peas
- 8 cups vegetable broth
- 1 cup coconut milk
- 1 medium onion, chopped
- 2 green onions, chopped
- 1/4 cup red bell pepper, diced
- 2 garlic cloves, minced
- 1 potato, cut in cubes
- 1 cup yam, dasheen, coco chopped, (optional)
- 1 carrot, diced
- 1 teaspoon dried thyme, or 2 sprigs of fresh
- 1 whole Scotch Bonnet pepper
- 6 pimento/allspice berries
- 1/2 teaspoon fresh ginger, grated
- 1 recipe Dumplings (visit website for recipe)
- sea salt, to taste
-

INSTRUCTIONS

1. Sort and wash beans, soak in water overnight or for at least 8 hours.

2. The following day, discard water and rinse beans, place them in a large saucepan with water and bring to boil, lower heat to simmer until tender for about 1 hour.

3. Add coconut milk, carrots, onion, garlic, and continue simmering. Add spinners and thyme and other seasonings, simmer for another 30 minutes or until sauce is thick. Discard pepper before serving. Delicious served with brown rice and a salad.

DUMPLINGS

1. Place flour and salt in a bowl. Add water and mix to make a stiff dough. Pinch off small pieces of dough and roll into the palm of hands to make long thin dumplings. Drop into simmering stew

 oh 40m   4

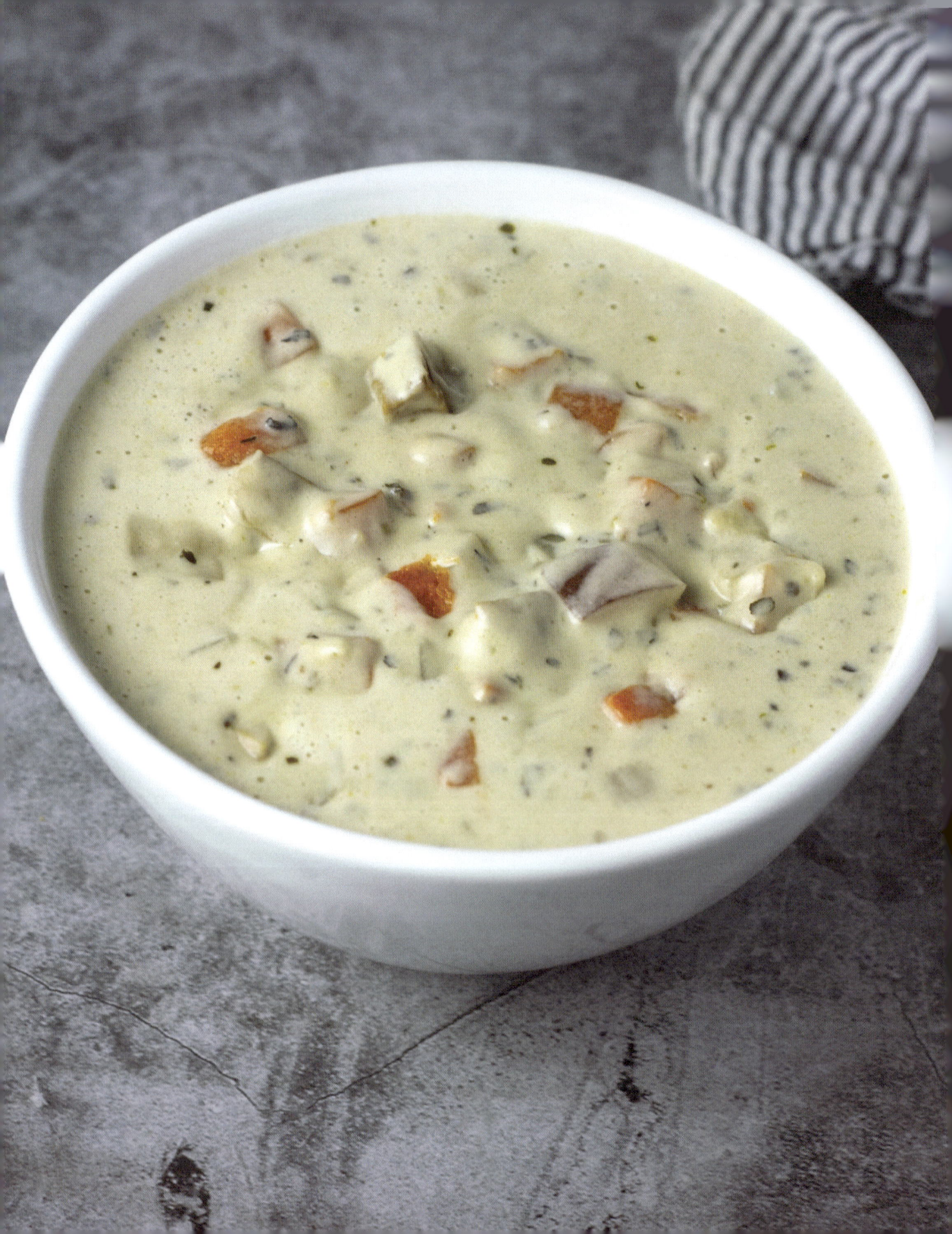

CREAM OF CHICKEN SOUP

Any chicken substitute of your choice can be used in this recipe, but I've included a simple tofu recipe that is so amazing in this soup. This soup is creamy comfort in a bowl.

INGREDIENTS

- 1 block of tofu, cut into small cubes
- 4 tablespoons nutritional yeast flakes
- 1 tablespoon liquid aminos or soy sauce
- 1 tablespoon Italian seasoning
- 2 teaspoons onion powder
- 1 teaspoon garlic powder
- 6 cups vegetable broth
- 2 cups onion, diced
- 4 carrots, diced
- 4 potatoes, diced
- 2 cups milk
- ¼ cup flour
- 1 cup milk
- ½ cup cashews

INSTRUCTIONS

1. Preheat oven to 350° F. Line a baking sheet with parchment paper or a silicone liner, and spray or brush with oil. In a bowl, add the tofu, yeast flakes, spices, and aminos.

2. Mix carefully with your hands. Spread out evenly on your baking sheet. Bake for 30-40 minutes, until tofu cubes are completely dry.

3. In a large pot on medium-high heat, add vegetable broth, onion, carrot, and potato, and bring to boil.

4. Bring heat to the lowest setting and allow to simmer until tofu comes out of the oven, 30 minutes.

5. Whisk flour and milk together, then add to soup and mix until fully incorporated. Add tofu and continue to simmer as the soup thickens.

6. Blend milk and cashews until fully smooth, and add to soup for that extra creaminess that makes this soup a luxury experience.

1h 30m   4

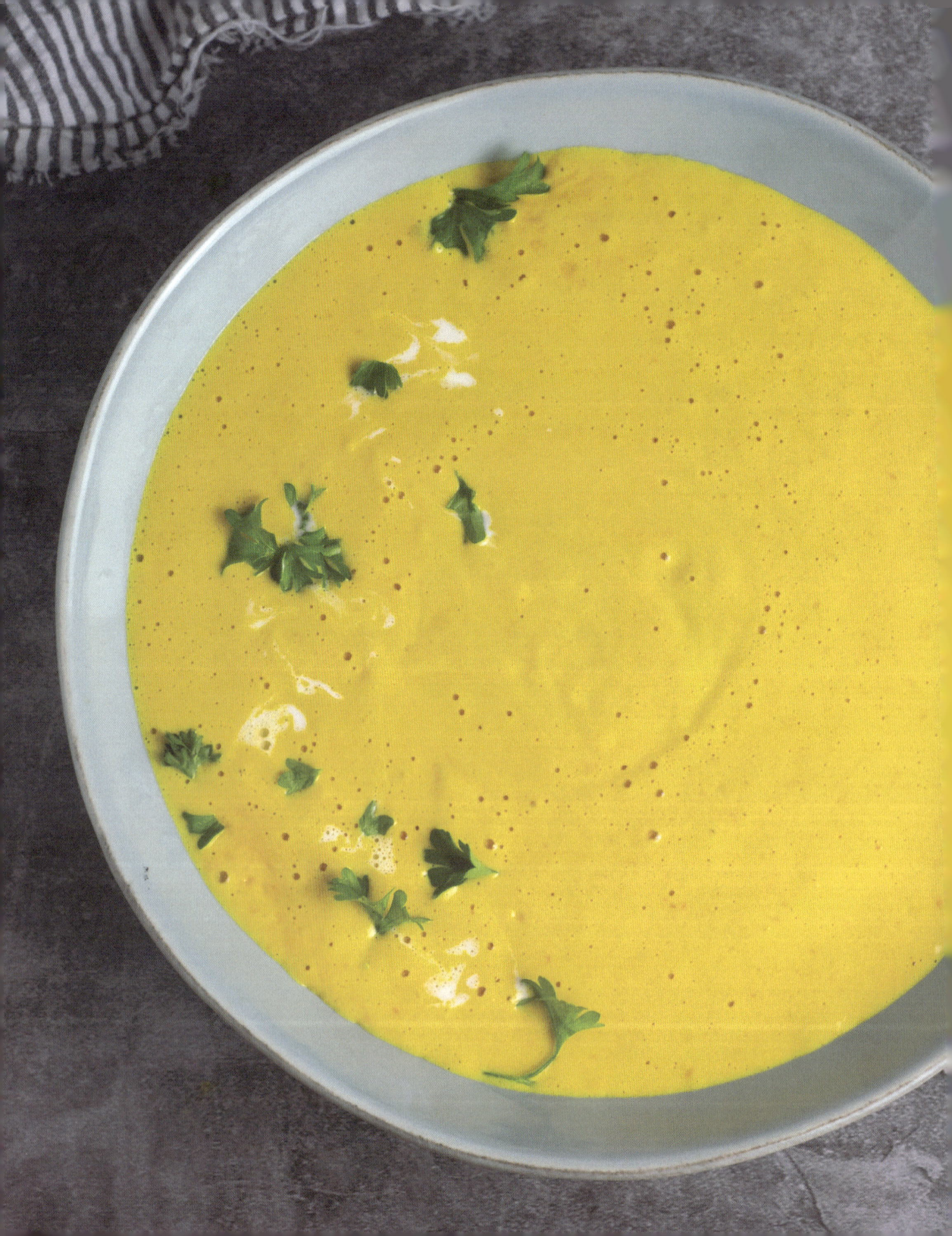

CURRIED BUTTERNUT SQUASH SOUP

Mildly sweet butternut squash is perfectly complemented by curry powder to make a mellow creamy soup with a kick of flavor.

INGREDIENTS

- 1 tablespoon coconut oil
- 1 cup onion, diced
- 4 cloves garlic, diced
- 6 cups diced butternut squash, fresh or frozen
- 2 tablespoons curry powder
- ½ teaspoon cumin
- ½ teaspoon coriander
- ¼ teaspoon salt
- 1/8 teaspoon cayenne
- 3 cups broth

INSTRUCTIONS

1. In a large pot, heat coconut oil on medium-low heat. Sauté onions until soft, about three minutes, then add garlic for two more minutes.

2. Add curry powder and other spices, and stir to coat onions and allow curry powder to fry, which brings out a delicious curry flavor without bitterness.

3. Add butternut squash, and coat in onion and spice mixture, then add vegetable broth and bring to boil. Lower heat and allow to simmer for 20 minutes, or when the squash is soft.

4. Blend in batches or with hand blender until fully pureed, and add more salt if necessary.

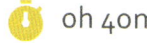 oh 40m   4

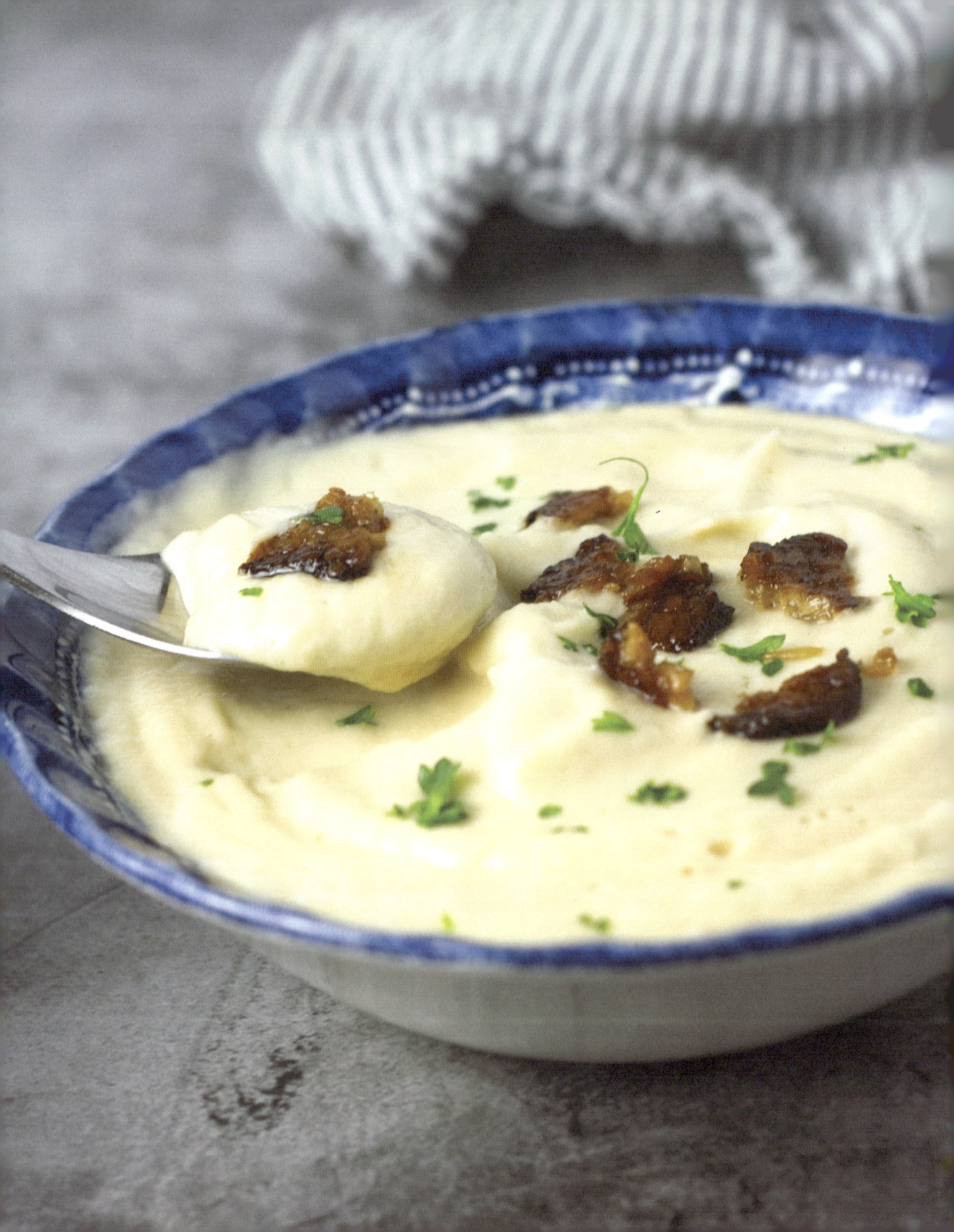

CREAMY CAULIFLOWER SOUP

Roasted cauliflower florets and garlic cloves makes this one of my favorite soups, with a wonderful smoky flavor, that is still so healthy.

INGREDIENTS

- 4-6 cups or one head of cauliflower florets, frozen or fresh
- 4 cloves garlic
- 1 tablespoon olive oil
- 1 cup onion, diced
- 4 cups vegetable broth
- 2 teaspoons Italian seasoning
- 1 teaspoon thyme
- 1 teaspoon oregano
- 1 teaspoon basil
- 1 tablespoon butter
- 1 teaspoon lemon
- salt, to taste
- **Garnishing ideas**
  - green onions
  - vegan cheddar cheese shreds
-

INSTRUCTIONS

1. Preheat your oven to 425° F.

2. On a parchment lined sheet pan, place cauliflower and garlic to roast on the top shelf of the oven for 25 minutes.

3. While they are roasting, in a large pot, heat olive oil on medium-low heat and sauté onions until soft, about three minutes.

4. Add vegetable broth and herbs, and bring to boil. Add cauliflower and garlic, bring heat to low, then simmer for 15 minutes.

5. Add butter and lemon to soup. Process until smooth in batches or with a hand blender, add salt if necessary.

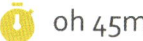 0h 45m   4

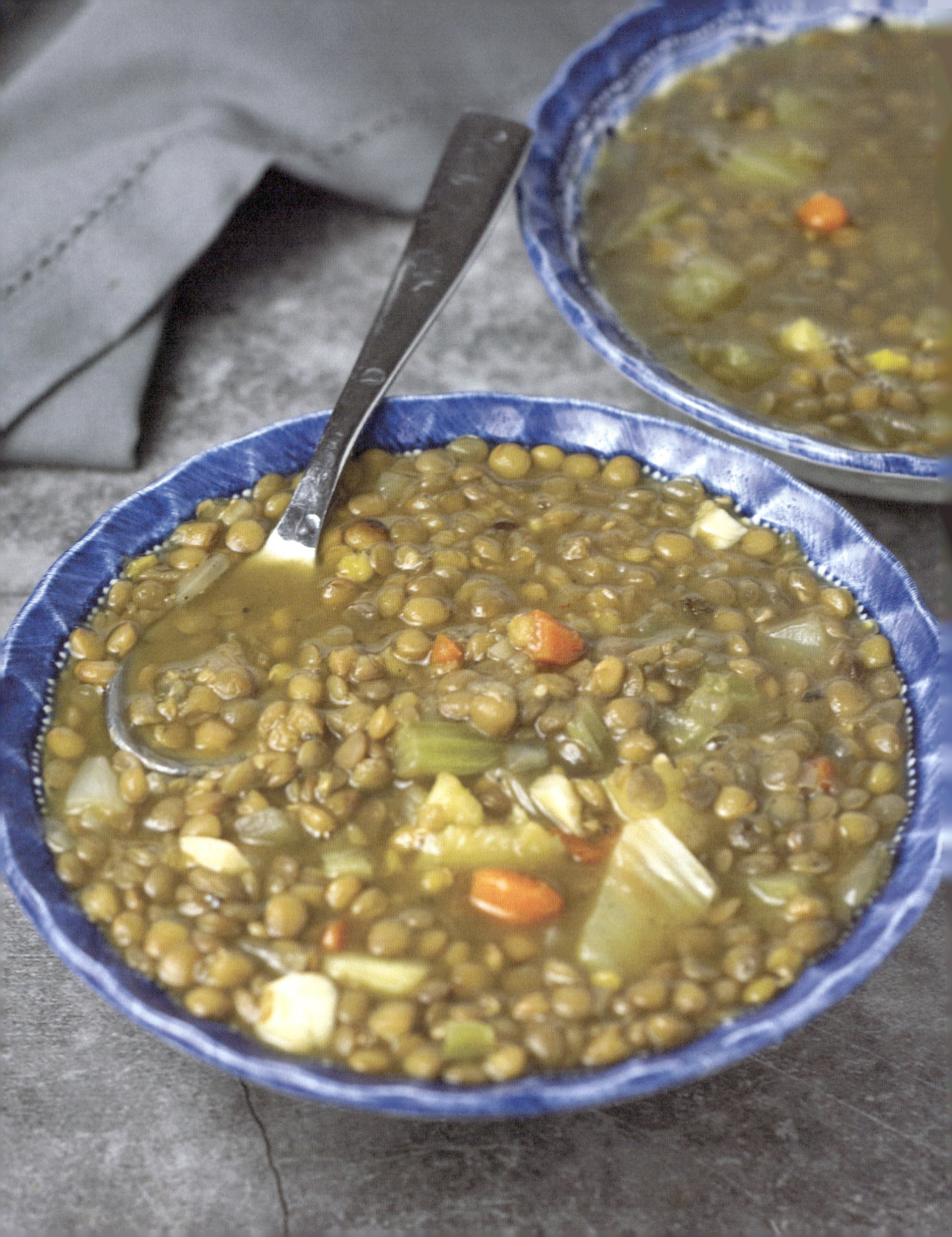

VEGAN LENTIL STEW

Hearty and flavorful Vegan Lentil Stew loaded with veggies, herbs and spices for a cozy and filling stew.

INGREDIENTS

- 1 1/2 cups dried lentils, green or brown lentils sorted and rinsed
- 1 tablespoon olive oil, or 1/4 cup water
- 1 medium onion, finely chopped
- 3 cloves garlic, minced
- 2 stalks celery, chopped
- 1 teaspoon Italian seasoning
- 1/2 teaspoon ground paprika
- 1/2 teaspoon cumin
- 1/2 teaspoon dried thyme
- 1 14 ounces can diced tomatoes
- 1 tablespoon tomato paste, (optional)
- 2 medium carrots, diced
- 1 medium potato, diced
- 6 cups vegetable broth
- 1 bay leaf
- 1/4 teaspoon Cayenne pepper
- salt, to taste
-

INSTRUCTIONS

1. Heat oil or water in a large saucepan over medium heat. Add onions and cook for about 3 minutes. Add garlic and cook for another minute

2. stir in celery, Italian seasoning, paprika, cumin and thyme and cook for 30 seconds.

3. Add lentils, tomatoes, tomato paste, carrots and potatoes, bay leaf and vegetable broth.

4. Bring to boil, reduce heat to simmer for about 40 minutes or until stew has reached the desired texture.

5. Remove bay leaf, season with salt and pepper and serve

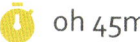 oh 45m   6

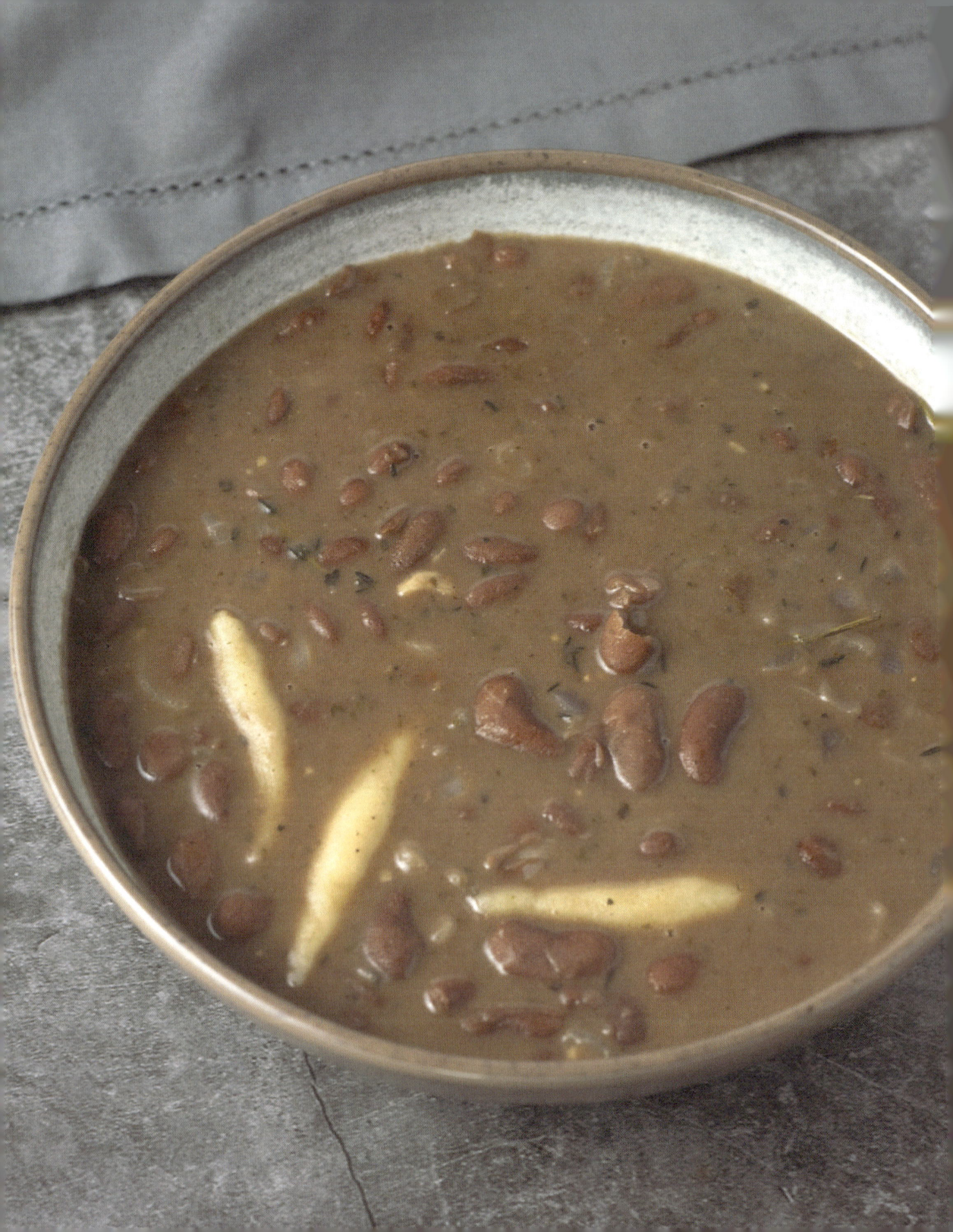

JAMAICAN STEW PEAS

Stew peas is a popular, tasty and hearty Jamaican dish. kidney beans also called red peas in Jamaica are cooked with flavorful coconut, aromatic spices, thyme, onion, garlic, and Scotch Bonnet pepper.

INGREDIENTS

- 2 cups dried kidney beans
- 6 cups water
- 1 14 ounce can coconut milk
- 1 medium onion, chopped
- 2 cloves garlic, minced
- 1 1/2 teaspoons salt, or to taste
- 1/2 teaspoon dried thyme, or 1 sprig of fresh
- 1 medium carrot, cut into coins
- 1 whole Scotch Bonnet pepper with stem intact
- 1/4 teaspoon fresh ginger, grated
- 1/4 teaspoon ground allspice or 6 berries
- 1 batch dumplings
- Dumplings
  - 1/2 cup flour, I used Krusteaz all-purpose flour
  - 1/4 cup cold water
  - 1/4 teaspoon salt

INSTRUCTIONS

1. Sort and wash beans, soak in water overnight or for at least 8 hours.

2. The following day, discard water and rinse beans, place them in a large saucepan with water and bring to boil, lower heat to simmer until tender for about 1 hour.

3. Add coconut milk, carrots, onion, garlic, and continue simmering. Add spinners and thyme and other seasonings, simmer for another 30 minutes or until sauce is thick. Discard pepper before serving. Delicious served with brown rice and a salad

DUMPLINGS

1. Place flour and salt in a bowl. Add water and mix to make a stiff dough. Pinch off small pieces of dough and roll into the palm of hands to make long thin dumplings. Drop into simmering stew.

1h 30m   4

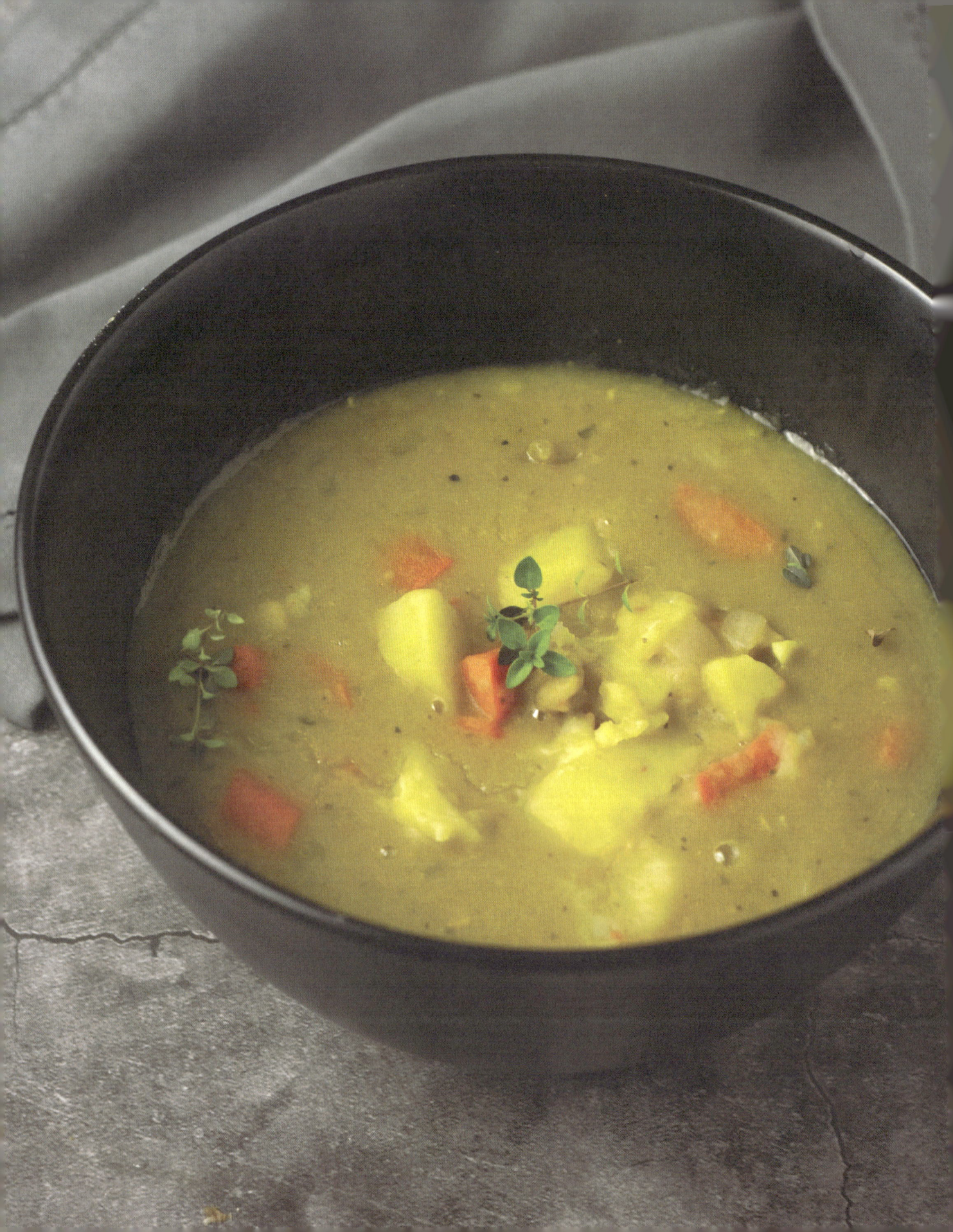

VEGAN SPLIT PEA SOUP

Simple and easy vegan split pea soup is so flavorful and hearty, perfect for cold nights but can be enjoyed all year. It is so economical, green split peas, carrots. potatoes, onion, garlic, cooked in vegetable broth.

INGREDIENTS

- 1 tablespoon coconut or olive oil
- 1 cup onion, chopped
- 2 cloves crushed garlic, minced
- 1 cup celery, chopped
- 1 teaspoon parsley flakes
- 1 sprig thyme, or 1/4 teaspoon dried thyme leaves
- 1/4 teaspoon dried oregano
- 1/2 teaspoon basil
- 1 bay leaf
- 1 carrot, chopped
- 1 medium potato, diced
- 2 cups green split peas, sorted and rinsed
- 7-8 cups vegetable broth
- sea salt, to taste
-

INSTRUCTIONS

1. Heat the oil in a large pot over medium heat. Cook onion, garlic and celery until onion is soft.

2. Stir in parsley, thyme, oregano, basil, and bay leaf, cook until fragrant.

3. Add carrot, potatoes, split peas, vegetable broth. Cover pot, and bring to boil.

4. Reduce to a simmer for one hour. Discard bay leaf and add salt to taste. Serve in a bowl.

 1h 15m   4

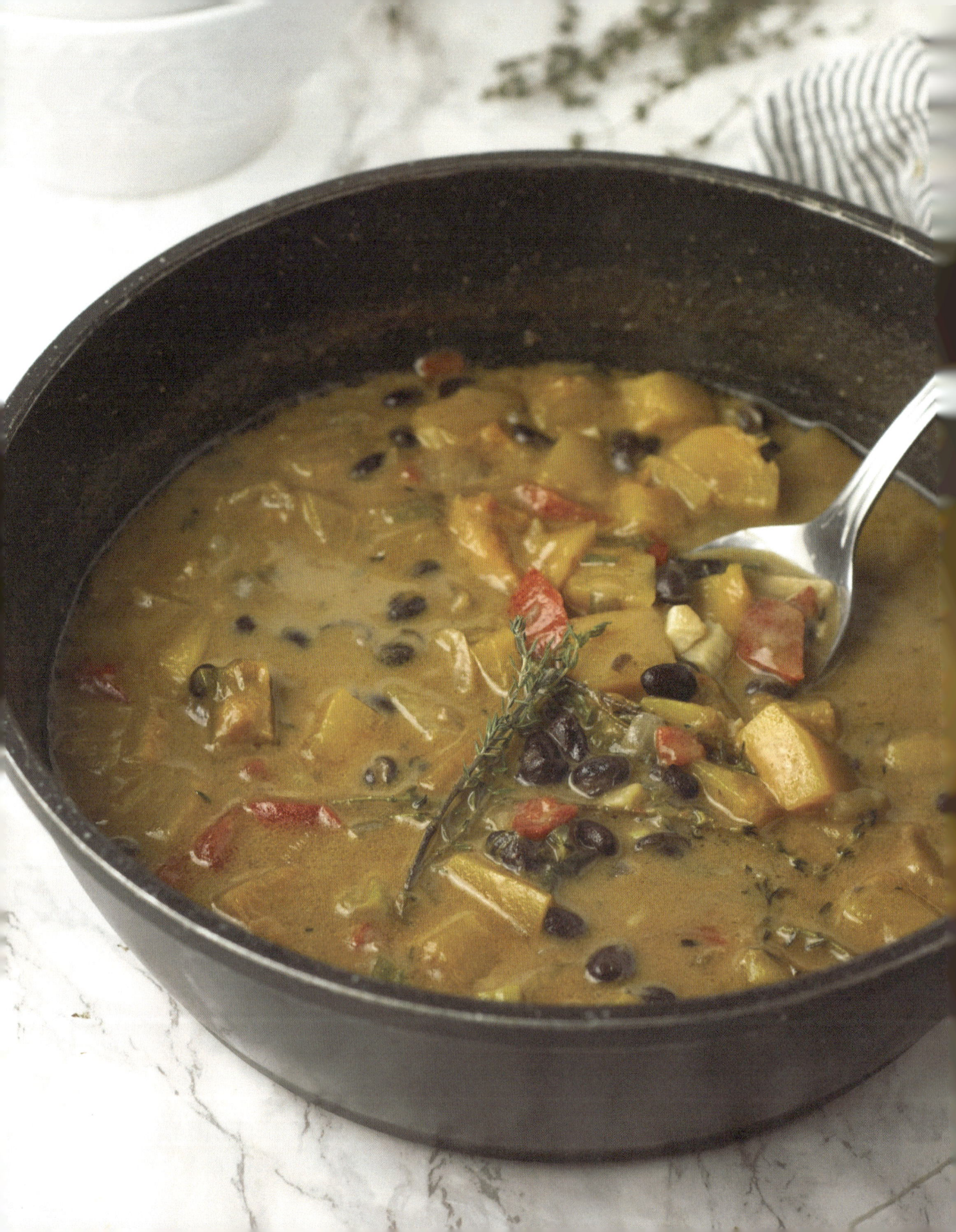

BLACK BEAN BUTTERNUT SQUASH STEW

Black bean with sweet butternut squash and collard greens make this healthy stew so hearty and comforting.

INGREDIENTS

- 1 tablespoon coconut oil
- 1 medium onion, chopped
- ½ medium red bell pepper, diced
- 3 cloves garlic, minced
- 2 green onions, chopped
- 2 cup butternut squash, peeled, and cut into ½ inch cubes
- 1 15 ounce can black beans, drained and rinsed
- ½ teaspoon Italian seasoning
- 2 sprigs thyme
- 1 cup coconut milk
- 1 cup vegetable broth
- 1 vegan bouillon, (I used Edward & Son's Not-Chick'n Bouillon Cubes)
- 1 cup tender collard greens, or kale or spinach, chopped (optional)
- ¼ teaspoon cayenne pepper
- pinch of allspice (optional)

INSTRUCTIONS

1. Heat the oil in a large pot over medium-high heat. Add onions and bell peppers, and cook until onions are soft, for about 3 minutes.

2. Stir in garlic and spring onion, and cook for one minute.

3. Add butternut squash, black beans, Italian seasoning, and thyme, and stir to coat.

4. Stir in coconut milk, vegetable broth, bouillon cube, allspice, and cayenne pepper.

5. Bring to a boil, then reduce heat to simmer for 20 minutes.

6. Stir in leafy greens and cook for about 4 minutes.

7. Eat in a bowl alone, or serve with brown rice and sliced avocado.

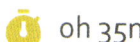 oh 35m 4

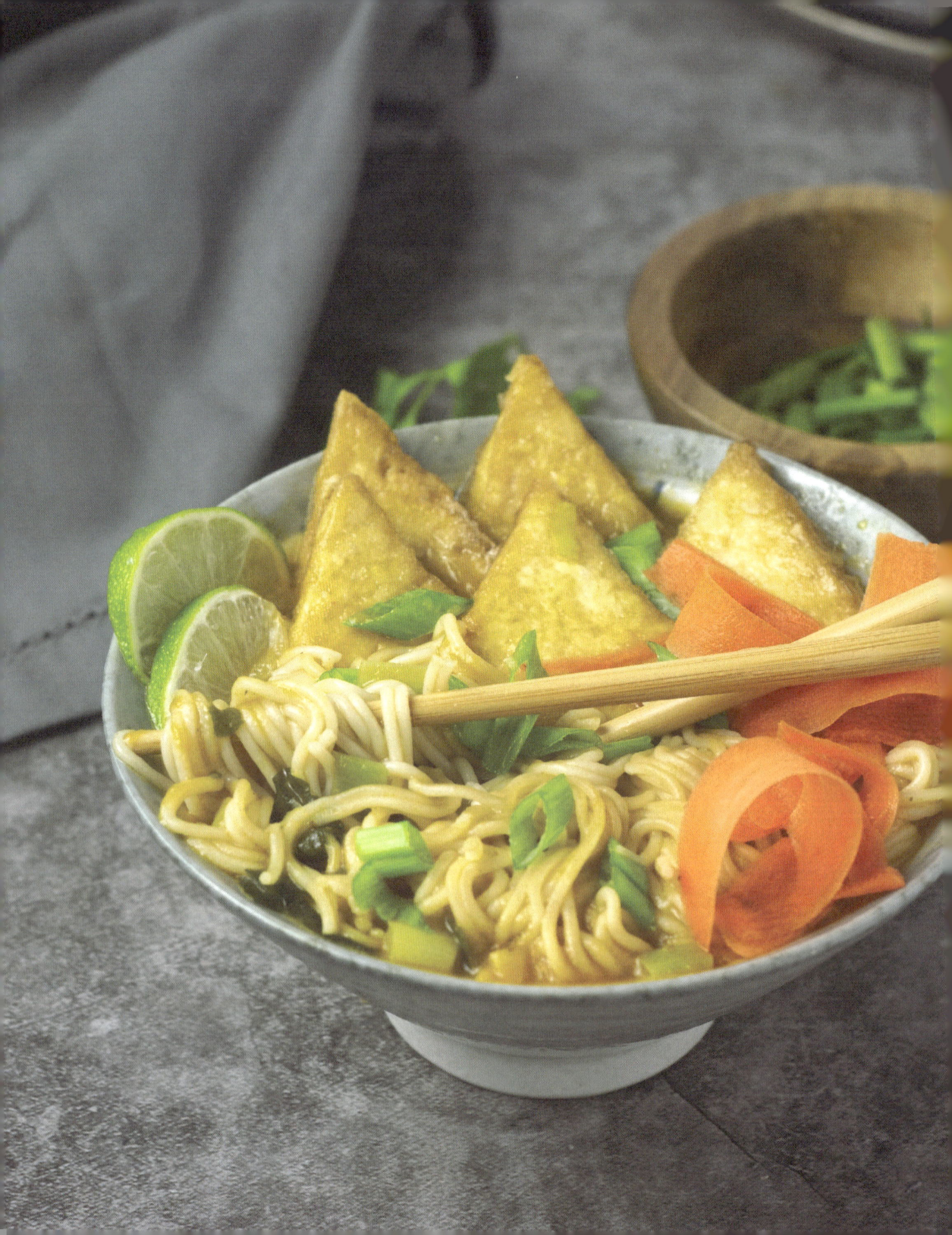

RAMEN

Enjoy this delicious vegan Ramen made from scratch in the comfort of your home, that simply amazing. Ramen noodles cooked in a flavorful homemade broth with carrots, onions, pepper, and aromatics topped with fried tofu and cilantro.

INGREDIENTS

- 4 ounces ramen noodles, (I used Lotus Foods Millet And Brown Rice Ramen)
- 1 tablespoon sesame oil
- 3 cloves garlic, minced
- 2 teaspoons fresh ginger, grated
- 1 stalk celery, finely chopped
- 2 green onions, finely chopped extra for garnish
- 2 sprigs thyme
- 1 medium carrot, shredded
- 3 cups vegetable broth
- 2 cups water
- 2-3 tablespoons Bragg's liquid aminos
- 2 tablespoon nutritional yeast flakes
- 1/4 teaspoon Cayenne pepper, (optional)
- Garnishing ideas
  - cilantro
  - green onion
  - carrot
  - red pepper

INSTRUCTIONS

1. Being that I was making this meatless ramen noodle soup, I had to boost the flavor by adding a few ingredients but the results were amazing, my son Daevyd ate half and wants me to make it again.

2. Press, drain tofu and cut into 1/4 inch slices. Place in a bowl and toss with Bragg's Liquid Aminos. Set aside to marinate.

3. Heat the oil in a large pot, add garlic, celery, ginger, green onion, thyme, and carrots.

4. Add vegetable broth, water, nutritional yeast flakes, Bragg's Liquid aminos, and bring to a boil. Reduce to a simmer for about 8 minutes.

5. Meanwhile, prepare the tofu, coat with cornstarch. Heat the oil in a large skillet and fry until golden and crisp on both sides. Remove from skillet and set aside.

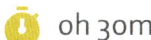 0h 30m 4

54

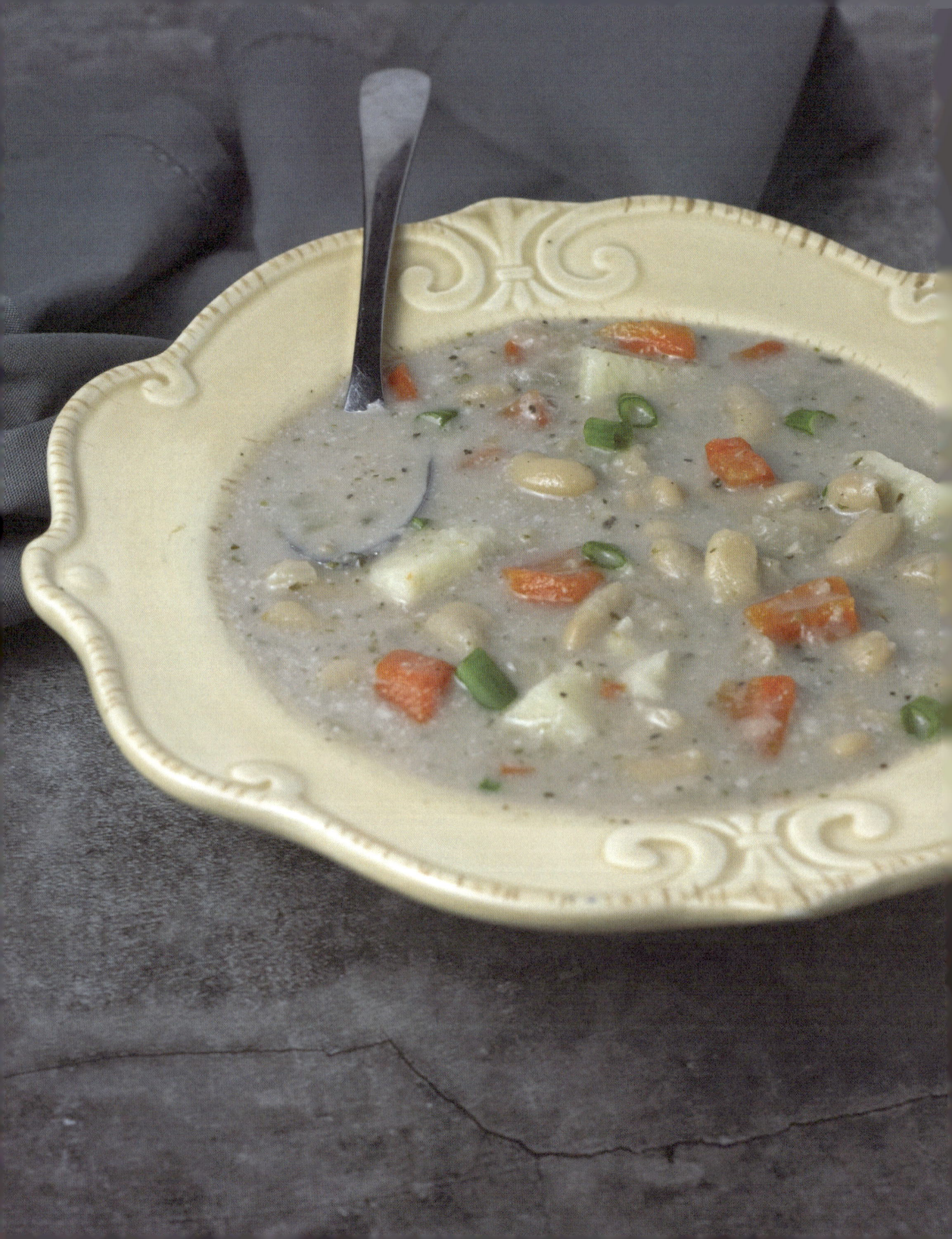

WHITE BEAN SOUP

Amazing Vegan White Bean Soup recipe that is hearty, comfy and full of flavor. It is vegan, gluten-free and oil-free and perfect for those long winter months.

INGREDIENTS

- 4 cups white beans, cooked or 8 oz dried (use Navy, Lima, Cannellini, Great Northern)
- 2 cups vegetable broth, or water
- 1 medium onion, chopped
- 2 cloves garlic, chopped
- 1 medium potato, diced
- 1 medium carrot, diced
- 1 teaspoon dried marjoram
- 1/2 teaspoon ground paprika
- 2 tablespoons coconut milk
- 1 teaspoon dried parsley flakes, or 2 teaspoon fresh leaves chopped
- 1/2 teaspoon dried thyme, or 1 sprig of fresh
- pinch of ground allspice
- 1 1/2 teaspoon salt, or to taste
- pinch of Cayenne pepper
- 1 bay leaf
- 1 tablespoon nutritional yeast flakes
-

INSTRUCTIONS

1. If you are using dried beans, prepare 8 oz of dried beans by sorting and washing.

2. Soak in water to cover for 8 hours or overnight. The following day, drain and rinse beans and cook in water until tender.

3. Place beans, water, onion, garlic, potato, carrot, marjoram, paprika, coconut milk, parsley, thyme, allspice, salt, cayenne pepper, bay leaf in a large pot.

4. Bring to a boil, and reduce to simmer for 30 minutes or until desired thickness is reached. Add yeast flakes, check the seasoning and serve immediately.

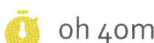 0h 40m   4

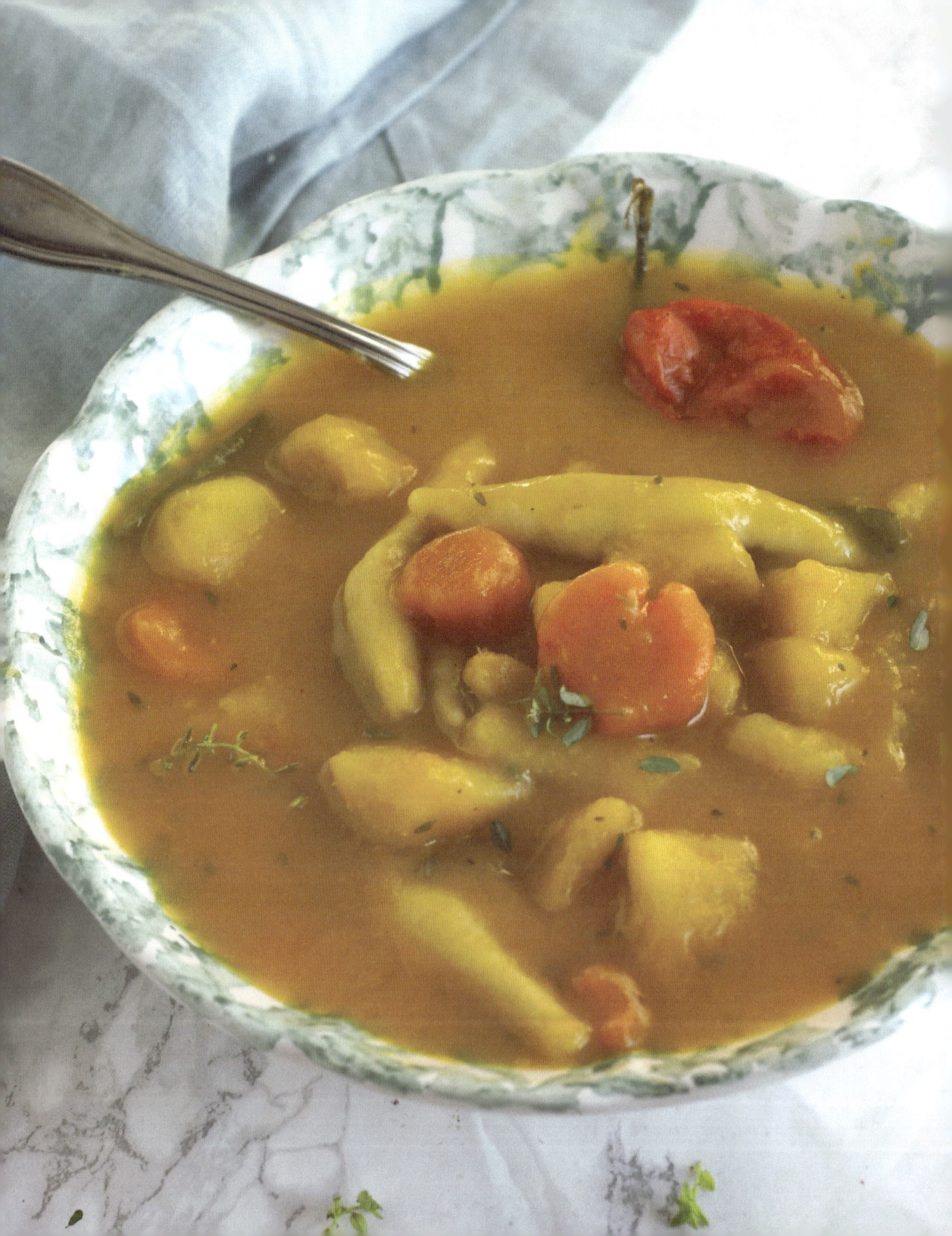

PUMPKIN SOUP WITH DUMPLINGS

This flavorful vegan pumpkin soup is an amazing Jamaican-style version. It has pumpkin, carrots, yellow yam, potato, chocho (chayote), and dumplings, cooked with a creamy, velvety and spicy coconut broth is perfect for Fall.

INGREDIENTS

- 4 cups pumpkin, peeled and chopped
- 6 cups vegetable broth
- 1 cup coconut milk
- 1 medium onion, chopped
- 3 cloves garlic, minced
- 2 green onions, chopped
- 1 medium white potato, peeled and cubed
- 2 stalks celery, chopped
- 1 medium carrot, chopped
- 1/4 teaspoon dried thyme
- 1/4 teaspoon allspice
- 1 Scotch Bonnet pepper
- salt, to taste
- Additional Vegetables
  - 1 pound yellow yam, or white yam, peeled and cubed
  - 1 medium chocho, peeled and chopped
- Dumplings
  - 1/4 cup water
  - 1/4 teaspoon salt
  - 1/2 cup all purpose gluten-free flour

INSTRUCTIONS

1. Bring vegetable broth to boil in a large pot, add pumpkin and cook until soft, about 10 minutes. Carefully mash pumpkin with a fork.

2. Add, coconut milk, onion, garlic, green onion, celery, carrot, potato, yam. Chocho, dumplings, thyme, allspice, dumplings and Scotch bonnet pepper on top of the soup. Cook for 20 minutes.

3. Note: Keep Scotch Bonnet Pepper whole, it is very hot if opened

DUMPLINGS

1. Combine flour and salt together in a mixing bowl.. Add enough water and mix with hands to form a stiff yet pliable dough. If it is too dry add water, if too soft add extra flour.

2. Pinch off a coin size piece of dough, roll between the palm of your hands to form a cylindrical shape dumpling. Repeat until finished. Add to the soup at least 15 minutes before it is finished cooking.

oh 45m   6

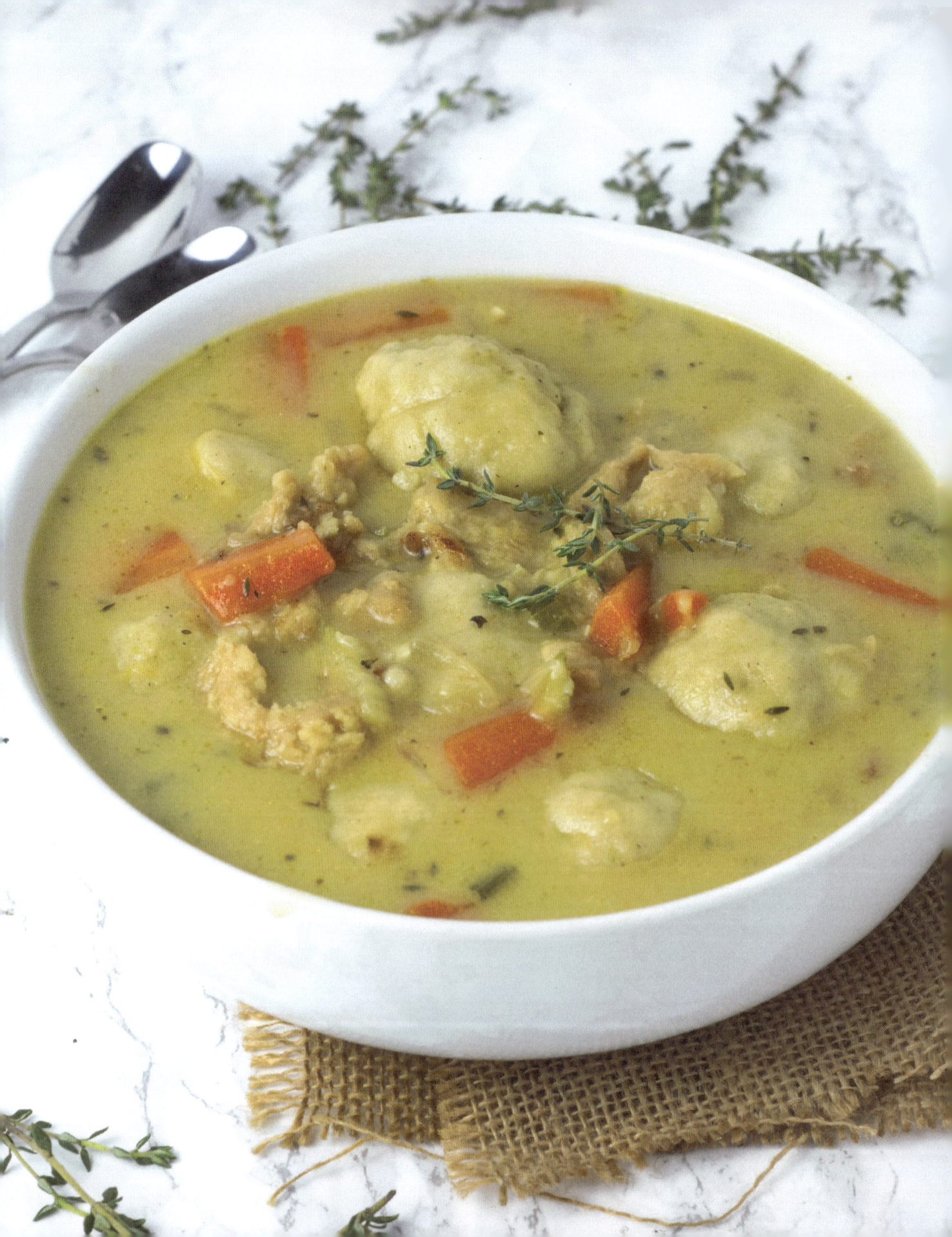

INSTANT POT VEGAN CHICKEN & DUMPLINGS

This amazing Instant Pot vegan chicken and dumplings is so easy to prepare, full of flavor with soy curls, soft fluffy gluten-free dumplings, carrots, celery, in a delicious broth.

INGREDIENTS

- Dumplings
  - 1 1/2 cups all purpose gluten-free flour
  - 2 teaspoons baking powder
  - 1/2 teaspoon salt
  - 2 tablespoons non-dairy butter,1 cup water
  - 1 tablespoon fresh parsley or chives, minced
- Soy Curls
  - 1 cup Butler Soy Curls™, soaked in boiling water for 10 minutes
  - 1 tablespoon Bragg's liquid aminos,
  - 1/2 teaspoon Italian seasoning
  - 2 tablespoons oil, (coconut, avocado, grape seed)
- Soup
  - 1 medium onion, chopped
  - 4 cloves garlic, chopped
  - 2 stalks celery, chopped
  - 2 medium carrots, peeled and chopped
  - 2 tablespoons all purpose gluten-free flour
  - 1/2 cup unsweetened almond milk
  - 4 cups vegetable broth
  - 1 teaspoon dried thyme leaves

- 2 tablespoons nutritional yeast flakes
- 1 bay leaf
- 1/2 teaspoon salt

INSTRUCTIONS

DUMPLINGS

1. Combine all-purpose gluten-free flour, baking powder, salt in a medium bowl.

2. Add butter and mix until crumbly, add water and parsley and mix to form a dough ball, set aside.

SOY CURLS

1. Drain soy curls and place them in a medium bowl. toss with Bragg's Liquid Aminos, and Italian Seasoning.

2. Select the Saute setting on the Instant Pot and heat the oil. It should say HOT. Add Soy Curls and cook stirring until starting to brown, about 3 minutes.

INSTANT POT VEGAN CHICKEN & DUMPLINGS

(CONTINUED)

SOY CURLS

1. Move the soy curls to one side of the Instant Pot, add onions, garlic, celery and cook stirring for 2 minutes.

2. Add carrots and stir. Move the vegetables leaving a spot and add the flour and cook for 1 minute.

3. Add almond milk, vegetable broth and de-glaze the bottom of the pot, using a wooden spatula to scrape the Instant Pot bottom.

4. Add thyme, nutritional yeast flakes, bay leaf, and salt. Divide the dumpling batter into 10 pieces, take each piece, roughly roll into a ball and drop on top of the soup and stir gently.

5. Secure the lid on the Instant Pot, turn the "Pressure Release" knob to the sealing position. Cancel the saute function. Press the "Pressure Cook/Manual" setting and set the cooking time for 5 minutes.

6. Let the pressure release naturally for 10 minutes, then move the pressure release to "Venting" to release the remaining steam. When the pin in the lid drops down, open the lid and stir, remove the bay leaf and serve.

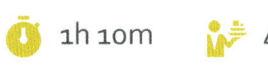 1h 10m   4

Printed in Great Britain
by Amazon